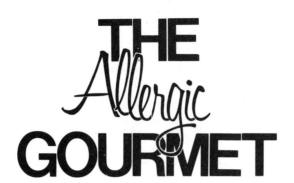

THE *Allergic* GOURMET

THE
Allergic
GOURMET

JUNE ROTH, M.S.

Contemporary Books, Inc.
Chicago

Library of Congress Cataloging in Publication Data

Roth, June Spiewak.
    The allergic gourmet.

    Includes index.
    1. Food allergy—Diet therapy—Recipes.   I. Title.
RC596.R66   1983   616.97′50654   83-1843
ISBN 0-8092-5612-6
ISBN 0-8092-5611-8 (pbk.)

Illustrations by Phil Kantz

First Contemporary trade paperback edition 1984

Published by Contemporary Books, Inc.
180 North Michigan Avenue, Chicago, Illinois 60601
Manufactured in the United States of America
Library of Congress Catalog Card Number: 83-1843
International Standard Book Number: 0-8092-5612-6 (cloth)
                                    0-8092-5611-8 (paper)

Published simultaneously in Canada by Beaverbooks, Ltd.
195 Allstate Parkway, Valleywood Business Park
Markham, Ontario L3R 4T8 Canada

Contents

To my dear friend Ruth Strauss, whose life is an example of courage and coping, turning adversity into adventure, while serving as an inspiration to all who are privileged to know and love her.

Foreword

Food sensitivities are responsible for much more than an occasional upset stomach or itching skin. Allergies often cause a variety of illnesses. Any organ of the body may be affected by food sensitivities, resulting in a disturbance in the function of that organ. When joints are affected, arthritis conditions may develop. When the lungs are the target of the allergy, coughs or asthma may be the result. When the nervous system is affected, the symptoms may be manifested as behavioral, mood, or thinking disorders.

Some may object to the use of the term *allergy*, because the mechanism producing the food sensitivity is not the same as that resulting in true allergic manifestations. This distinction may be important to scientists and physicians, but to the individual who suffers because a particular food causes a severe reaction, the distinction is purely academic. *Food sensitivities* and *food allergies* are used interchangeably for the purposes of this discussion.

Physicians are recognizing that frequent exposure to the same food often results in a sensitivity to that food. Think of how often our meals and snacks include dairy products, eggs, and flour—it is not unusual to find these foods eaten two or three times a day. When individuals are tested for allergies a majority of them reveal sensitivities to these common ingredients. There is often great difficulty in removing one or more of these foods from the diet, unless one is a skilled cook. June Roth, in her excellently written *The Allergic Gourmet,* makes it easy for the patient to learn how to cope with restrictions. She takes into account those foods that cause sensitivities most often—dairy products, eggs, and the gluten flours. And then, recognizing that multiple allergies are often present, she adds a section for those who suffer from all three of the major sensitivities. The problem of obtaining the proper nutrients from food while on a restricted diet is also discussed, and a few easy-to-follow rules are outlined to ensure good nutrition.

When starting a diet for allergies, which usually is a list of "thou shalt nots," the average person becomes overwhelmed and quite discouraged. The usual comment is, "I can't go on this diet. There is nothing left to eat." *The Allergic Gourmet* silences forever that familiar complaint. Even better, the author has made possible what has only been dreamt of before: to be allergic and not be deprived of the gourmet experience. Thank you, June Roth!

Harvey M. Ross, M.D.
President, The International College of Applied Nutrition
President, The Academy of Orthomolecular Psychiatry

DEAR READER,

According to thousands of letters sent to me by readers of my syndicated newspaper column "Special Diets," one of the most difficult of all cooking problems is coping with the elimination of a food staple from the diet. The letters resound with feelings of frustration in attempting to make marketing habits, cooking techniques, and menu planning conform to a prescription to avoid milk products, eggs, or wheat and all of its related gluten flours. My impression is that most of my correspondents are limiting their meals and cooking talents, rather than expanding the menus into a wider realm of food possibilities.

This is not to make light of a food restriction because of an existing allergy or malabsorption problem, but to face up to it and to learn how to have an adventurous palate without the offending food. Yes, even to learn how to cook gourmet meals, bake bread and cookies without wheat flour, and enjoy as many gustatory pleasures as can be devised within the limitations.

I have been longing to write this book to show you how to cope in the allergic person's kitchen. Perhaps you will be inspired to triumph over what seems to be an impossible food elimination problem and to become a better cook than ever before.

I shall be cheering you on!

Warmly,

June Roth

1
How to Cope with Food Allergies

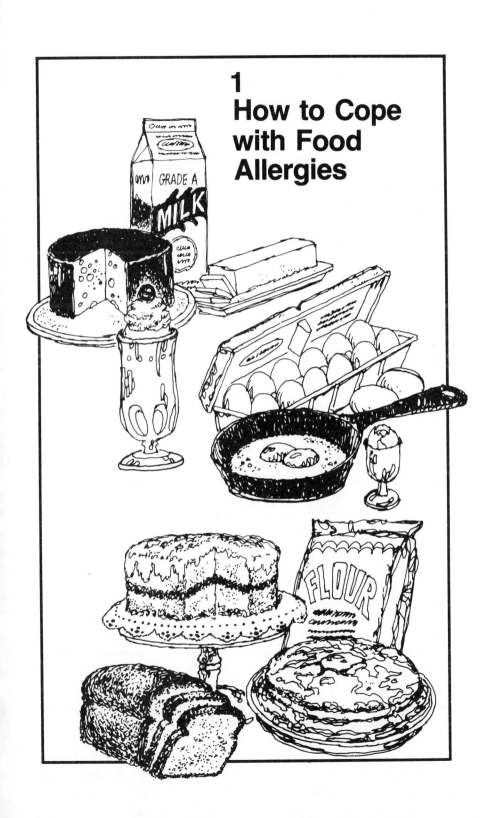

If you thought that you would never have food allergies and you are feeling inept and discouraged in the face of eliminating the food that is causing you trouble, join the club. The club is ever growing and consists of people who have been made aware of their (or a family member's) sensitivities to certain foods that seem to cause mood swings, stomach upsets, or rashes. As medical practitioners become more adept at diagnosing these sensitivities and eliminating the need to mask the symptoms with medication, more and more individuals are suddenly thrust into a quandary concerning how to cope with restrictions.

It's normal to feel hopeless and helpless when first confronted with the fact that you or someone you love is going to have to subtract a certain food or group of foods from the diet. Perhaps this change will be permanent, and perhaps not, as some food sensitivities are often outgrown or replaced with new ones.

What's the cook to do?

It makes good sense to approach the problem optimistically, to see the water glass as half full rather than half empty. Concentrate on all the good that is present, not on what is missing. Make a list of all the foods that *can* be eaten and plan your menus from that list.

Now make another list of foods that you (or the person you're cooking for) do not usually eat because of ethnic habits, an unadventurous spirit, or routine meal planning. Start to introduce some of these foods into the menus so that something interesting is happening to the meals while a food is being eliminated.

If the food to be eliminated is one kind of vegetable, shellfish, or a group of fruits, you will probably find the allergy fairly simple to deal with. However, if the food is one or more of the three staple elements of most kitchen preparation—dairy products, eggs, or gluten flours—you may have to invest a little more time and thought into meal planning to keep your menus interesting. But it *can* be done. In fact, with the help of this book, which has done a major part of the thinking for you in devising allergen-free recipes, you can do this with ease.

There are other sensitivities that do not have an entire section of recipes devoted to them in this book, but you will find helpful hints for dealing with these allergies throughout the book. These allergies include corn, potatoes, and chocolate.

It is a simple matter to avoid corn on the cob and not to use cornstarch when a sensitivity to corn exists. But one must also watch out for products that contain corn oil, corn syrup, dextrose (glucose), hominy, grits, and popped corn. Although you may not cook with it, cornstarch is a thickener that is found in many foods such as catsup, Chinese dishes, cough syrups, ice creams, pastas, creamed pies, and cakes. You'll have to be particularly vigilant to eliminate contact with corn, as subsidiary products are used in many of the items we use everyday. Corn products can be found in such surprising places as the adhesives used on stamps and envelopes, the composition of paper cups and plates, talcum powder, and vitamin pills.

Some people are sensitive to potatoes, and it is necessary to read labels carefully to be sure that potato starch has not been used as a thickening agent in a manufactured food product. Besides eliminating the use of potatoes, be suspicious of vegetable soups and mixed vegetables.

For most other food sensitivities, it is possible to simply eliminate the offending ingredient from your diet. When allergic to chocolate, you might want to occasionally use carob. Nuts are all from different genuses, so it's worth your while to establish which nuts are causing the problems and thus be able to eat those that test out all right for you. If you have a sensitivity to beets, be aware that beet sugar is often used in manufactured food products and that you will have to do some detecting to be sure you are not eating what will give you unwanted reactions.

It's always best to do your own cooking to be able to eliminate an allergen, or to choose very simple cooked to order foods when dining out. When you do order food in a restaurant, choose items that can be prepared to order rather than those that may have a processed product as the base or that may be sauced to a point at which you can't recognize possible ingredient allergens.

In this book, the recipe sections are divided into four groups. The first group is for the person who must eliminate dairy products. The second is geared to egg-free cooking. The third group shows how to deal with alternative flour possibilities when eliminating wheat and its related gluten flours. This gluten-free section also contains an alternate flour substitution list and suggestions for experimenting with some of your favorite recipes to try to convert them into allergen-free recipes. In the final section, a combination of all three sensitivities is confronted with amazingly delicious results.

Be sure to note that in each individual allergy section suggestions are often given for changing recipes to compensate for multiple allergies as well. In the dairy-free section, for instance, if a recipe is also egg-free or gluten-free, it is so marked. If there is a way to change a recipe to make it egg-free, for example, that possibility will be noted in the introduction to the recipe.

This method is followed in each of the specialized allergy sections, so that the person in need of dairy-free/egg-free recipes but who can have wheat flour will find a group of recipes that will meet those needs. Other combinations will be offered in the same manner, so look at the clues at the start of each recipe to determine whether that recipe will fit your particular cooking needs. So do take time to browse through all of the recipe sections; the recipes have been divided for easy reference but can be valuable to you in many ways.

Each recipe section will give you advice about how to ferret out hidden no-no's in the prepared food supply. Mostly it is a matter of learning how to read labels. Make it a practice to avoid foods that have a wide assortment of chemicals on the label—processed foods. Allergic people may also have a sensitivity to one or more of these chemicals. For these reasons, you will find certain ingredients listed in recipes as "pure." This is to alert you to the fact that certain brands or types of this ingredient contain potential allergens, so be a wary buyer of ingredients such as soy sauce or Worcestershire sauce.

Notice that many of the recipes make use of a variety of herbs and spices, vinegar, wine, lemon, garlic, onion, and other flavor enhancers. You are going to be a better cook when you season foods better, and hopefully the allergic person in your household is going to be eating better and feeling better than ever before. You will find that if you depend on fresh fruit and vegetables, start-from-scratch recipes, and simple broiled meats, poultry, and fish, you will be able to cope admirably with any restriction—even the triple whammy of the dairy-free/egg-free/gluten-free diet!

For additional variety and interesting dishes, visit several different kinds of ethnic grocery stores. For instance, Chinese markets offer many rice products that may not be available in your supermarket. They are not as expensive to purchase as those in health food stores and will suit your needs if you must avoid wheat and gluten products. One of these items is noodles made from rice. Another is rice crackers—crispy and enjoyable for someone who can't have wheat crackers and yearns for a nibble or dipper. Ethnic markets catering to a Spanish-speaking clientele have a variety of cornmeal products featuring fine-to-coarse grind meal, tapioca, many interesting dried beans, and an assortment of intriguing fruits and vegetables.

New foods are advisable for the allergic as variety in the menu will prevent boredom and will also provide foods to which a sensitivity has not been acquired. Introduce them one at a time to be sure there is no reaction and rotate them into the diet so that the chances for building up a sensitivity will be reduced. Chapters 2 and 3 will show you the wisest way to plan good nutritious menus for the entire family, but especially for some-one who may be sensitive to a food that is essential to growth and development. You will learn about the relationship that foods have with each other; for example, they belong to families that may also have to be eliminated when one member of the food family provokes an allergic response.

We have designed a special index to this book so that you can easily determine the content of each recipe. In this index, each recipe is carefully marked as to whether it is dairy-free (DF), egg-free (EF), and/or gluten-free (GF). For additional details on how to use the index, see page 277.

What you will not find in this book are silly food tricks to make up for the restrictions. If a dairy-free soup can have a creamy appearance, you'll find a recipe for it without milk. If it can't, then you will be able to choose from a variety of other recipes. The promise is that you will have a wide selection of excellent food despite having major allergies to consider during food preparation. Sometimes it is better just to eliminate a particular food from the diet than to stir up false hopes and faulty tastes. Therefore, do not expect to find recipes for mock cheese, mock eggs, or mock pizza. Let's be honest about the food sensitivities that exist and the best ways to cope and still have excellent food.

So browse among hundreds of delicious recipes that are care-fully marked to help you choose wisely for the person with a food sensitivity. The recipes are designed to appeal to everyone in the household, making it possible to cook the same meal for all.

2
Planning
Nutritious
Menus

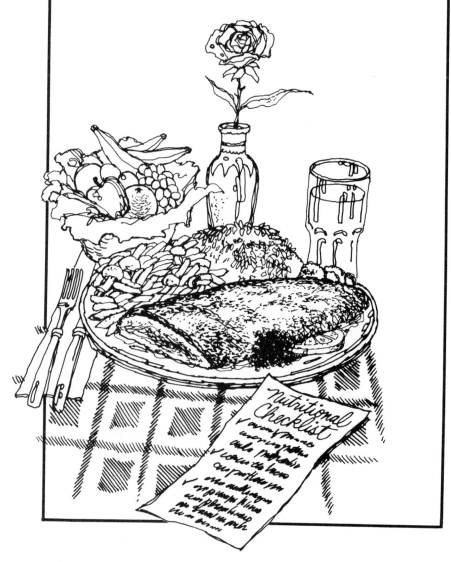

Every member of the household is entitled to good health. Good health starts with good nutrition, which in turn is based on a balance of protein, carbohydrates, and fats, along with essential vitamins and minerals. There is an art to working all of these into a daily meal plan to keep the food attractive and tasty, and to selecting ingredients that are of high-density nutrient value, supplying optimal nutrition with every calorie.

Our foods have been divided into four food groups. These make it easier to remember to include some of each in the menu planning. Here is a recommended way to pattern foods from these groups:

THE MEAT GROUP

Eat two or more servings a day of meat, poultry, fish, eggs, dried beans, dried peas, lentils, or peanut butter. Each of the following is considered one serving.

2–3 ounces of boneless meat, poultry, or fish
2 eggs
1 cup cooked dried beans, dried peas, or lentils
4 tablespoons peanut butter

THE MILK GROUP

Eat two or more eight-ounce servings of milk a day. Part or all of the milk may be skim milk, buttermilk, evaporated milk, or dry milk. Substitutions for milk may be made as follows.

1-inch wedge cheddar cheese = ½ cup (4 ounces) milk
½ cup cottage cheese = ⅓ cup (3 ounces) milk
2 tablespoons cream cheese = 1 tablespoon milk
½ cup ice cream = ¼ cup (2 ounces) milk

THE VEGETABLE-FRUIT GROUP

Eat four or more servings (one serving is generally ¹/₂ cup or one whole fruit) a day of fruits and vegetables.

Choose one serving of fruits or vegetables from the vitamin A list (below) at least every other day. To help you remember them, notice that these foods are all dark green or dark yellow in color.

Choose one serving of citrus fruit or juice from the vitamin C list (below) every day and choose one serving of vegetables from the vitamin C list every day. (Note that some fruits and vegetables contain both vitamin A and vitamin C.)

For the remaining serving(s) you can either make your own choice of fruits and vegetables, or use extra servings from the following vitamin A and C lists.

Vitamin A Fruits

Apricots
Cantaloupe
Mangoes
Persimmons

Vitamin A Vegetables

Broccoli
Carrots
Chard
Collards
Cress
Kale
Pumpkin
Spinach
Sweet potatoes
Turnip greens
Winter squash

Vitamin C Fruits

Grapefruit
Guava
Honeydew melon
Lemons
Mangoes
Oranges
Papaya
Strawberries
Tangerines
Watermelon

Vitamin C Vegetables

Asparagus
Broccoli
Brussels sprouts
Cabbage
Collards
Cress
Green pepper
Kale
Kohlrabi
Mustard greens
Potatoes and sweet potatoes
  cooked in their jackets
Spinach
Sweet red peppers
Tomatoes
Turnip greens

THE BREAD-CEREAL GROUP

Eat four or more servings a day. Each of the following is considered one serving.

1 slice bread
1 ounce ready-to-eat cereal
½ cup cooked cereal, cornmeal, grits, macaroni, noodles, rice, or spaghetti

THE DAILY DOZEN

A simple way to remember these four food groups during your menu planning is to calculate them as your daily dozen.

2 servings of the Meat Group
2 servings of the Milk Group
4 servings of the Vegetable-Fruit Group
4 servings of the Bread-Cereal Group

VITAMINS IN YOUR FOOD

Vitamin A

Vitamin A is found in whole milk, butter, eggs, leafy green and yellow vegetables and fruits, and liver. Vitamin A is essential to developing and maintaining healthy eyes, skin, hair, teeth, and gums, and is also involved in fat metabolism.

Vitamin B₁

Vitamin B_1 is found in whole-grain or enriched bread and cereals, yeast, liver, pork, fish, lean meat, poultry, milk, and legumes. Vitamin B_1 liberates energy from food and is necessary to proper function of the heart and nervous system.

Vitamin B₂

Vitamin B_2 is found in milk, whole-grain or enriched bread and cereals, liver, lean meat, eggs, and leafy green vegetables. Vitamin B_2 facilitates the body's use of carbohydrates, proteins, and fats, particularly for providing energy to cells, and is needed for healthy tissue.

Vitamin B6

Vitamin B6 is found in lean meats, leafy green vegetables, whole-grain cereals, dried yeast, and bananas. Vitamin B6 is important in metabolism, in the synthesis of proteins, in the use of fats, and in the formation of red blood cells.

Vitamin B12

Vitamin B12 is found in liver, kidney, fish, milk, and other foods of animal origin. Vitamin B12 helps build nucleic acids for the cell nucleus and to form red blood cells. It is an important aid in the functioning of the nervous system.

Vitamin C

Vitamin C is found mainly in citrus fruits, other fruits, tomatoes, leafy green vegetables, and potatoes. Vitamin C helps keep bones, teeth, and blood vessels healthy and is important in the formation of collagen, which helps support the body skeleton.

Vitamin D

Vitamin D is found in fortified milk, cod liver oil, egg yolks, tuna, and salmon. Vitamin D is needed for strong teeth and bones and helps the body use its calcium and phosphorus supply properly.

Vitamin E

Vitamin E is found in vegetable oils, whole-grain cereals, wheat germ, and lettuce. Vitamin E helps in the formation and functioning of red blood cells, muscle and other tissues, and protects essential fatty acids.

Vitamin K

Vitamin K is found in leafy green vegetables. Vitamin K is required for normal blood clotting.

MINERALS IN YOUR FOOD

Iron

Iron is found in liver, other meats, eggs, dried beans and

peas, green leafy vegetables, prunes, raisins, dried apricots, and enriched or whole-grain breads and cereals. Iron combines with protein to make hemoglobin and to carry oxygen to cells and is part of important enzymes.

Calcium

Calcium is found in milk, cheese, fortified cereals, broccoli, kale, collards, and turnip greens. Calcium helps build bones and teeth, helps keep muscles and nerves healthy, helps blood clot, and helps regulate the body's use of other minerals.

Phosphorus

Phosphorus is found in liver, fish, poultry, eggs, cheese, milk, whole-grain cereals, and nuts. Phosphorus is essential in building bones and teeth, in releasing energy, and in muscle and nerve function.

Iodine

Iodine is found in seafood, in plants grown in soil near the sea, and in iodized salt. Iodine forms part of the hormones produced by the thyroid to help regulate metabolism.

Copper

Copper is found in nuts, raisins, liver, kidney, some shellfish, and mushrooms. Copper is present in many organs, such as the brain, liver, heart, and kidneys, as part of the proteins and enzymes involved in brain and red cell function.

Magnesium

Magnesium is found in red meat, potatoes, nuts, corn, green leafy vegetables, and whole-grain or fortified cereals. Magnesium is an important part of all soft tissues and bones and helps trigger many vital enzyme reactions.

Zinc

Zinc is found in red meat, liver, eggs, seafood, milk, and whole-grain products. Zinc is essential for normal skeletal growth and tissue repair and is part of several important hormones, including insulin.

Trace Metals

Chromium, manganese, molybdenum, selenium, and fluorine are trace metals, and they are found in red meats, cereals, nuts, fruits, and vegetables. Trace metals are needed in a wide variety of normal body functions. Fluorine, for example, makes teeth harder. Chromium is involved in the metabolism of glucose into energy. Manganese activates enzymes and helps to maintain sex-hormone production. Molybdenum may prevent anemia, and selenium preserves tissue elasticity and may prevent premature aging.

PROTEIN, CARBOHYDRATES, AND FAT

Protein

Protein is found in meat, fish, poultry, eggs, milk, cheese, dried beans, dried peas, peanut butter, nuts, breads, and cereals. Protein helps build and repair all tissues, helps build blood, and helps form antibodies to fight infection. Protein supplies energy.

Carbohydrates

Carbohydrates are found in breads, cereals, pastas, potatoes, lima beans, corn, dried beans, dried peas, dried fruits, sweetened fruits, sugars, syrups, jellies, jams, and honey. It can also be made in the body from protein. Carbohydrates supply energy, carry other nutrients present in foods, and supply bulk.

Fat

Fat is found in butter, cream, most cheeses, salad oils and dressings, egg yolks, cooking fats, fat in meat. Fat supplies large amounts of energy through a small amount of food; supplies essential fatty acids; carries fat-soluble vitamins A, D, E, and K; protects vital organs; and is a building block for hormones.

PLANNING BALANCED MENUS

When planning menus, be sure to include the basic four food groups in the form of the daily dozen. Consider the vitamins, minerals, protein, carbohydrates, and fat that should be part of each day's menus—write everything down, rather than catch meals on the run while hoping that you have eaten a balanced diet.

Determine how many calories you need to maintain your best weight. The best health plan is to try to limit protein intake to 12% of the daily calories, limit fat to 30% or less, and increase the amount of complex carbohydrates—vegetables, fruits, whole grained breads and cereals. Lower the amount of simple sugar in the diet, including not only table sugar but also syrups, honey, brown sugar, and molasses.

With these goals in mind, work all food restrictions into this basic plan, and you will find that there are many good food substitutions that will give you a satisfactory range of meal choices while also giving you a healthy diet despite allergies.

There is an art to eating well and feeling well. It all starts with balanced menu planning.

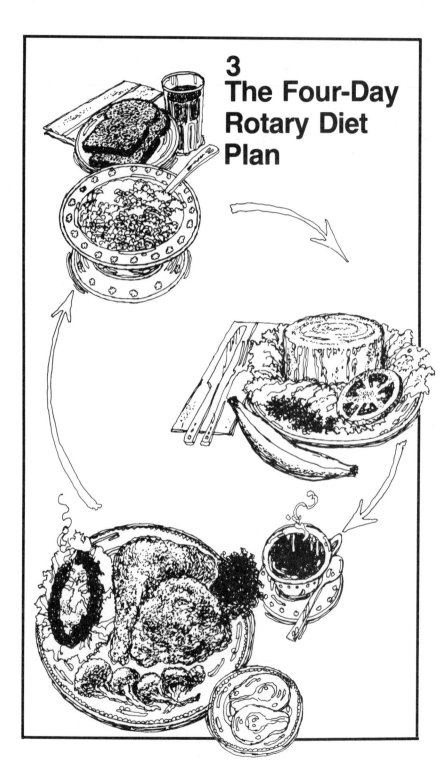

3
The Four-Day Rotary Diet Plan

There are times when a physician will advise an allergic patient to follow a four-day rotary diet. This means that when a food is eaten, it cannot be eaten again until four days have passed. (Already-known allergens, of course, are not included on the rotary diet menu plan.) It's the kind of prescription that can cause havoc in the kitchen. It is recommended when a patient displays a wide variety of food allergies and for those who seem to pick up new ones with regularity.

The rotary diet is often prescribed for a short period of time, such as several weeks, to determine whether any particular meal has caused a reaction. If it has, you can easily isolate the ingredients in that meal by serving them one at a time to retest them and pinpoint the food that is causing the problem.

This plan is also used as a way of giving the body a rest from doses of addictive foods, because allergic people often reach for just the foods that are causing them problems frequently throughout each day. For example, a child who has hyperactive behavior bouts after drinking cow's milk often drinks large quantities of milk all day long, getting a "fix" much as an addict would. When that food occurs on the menu only once in four days, the child is likely to crave it, revealing the milk as a likely allergen. Avoiding frequent repetition of any food through the rotary diet lessens the potential for developing new food sensitivities for those who exhibit this pattern. Transit time (the period between eating a food and eliminating the wastes from it) is between 18 and 24 hours, so the four-day rotary method gives foods plenty of time to leave the body before the same type of food is eaten again.

FOOD FAMILIES AND THE ROTARY DIET

Foods that are related, such as the cabbage family of broccoli, Brussels sprouts, and kohlrabi, may be placed on the menu two days apart. This means, for instance, that if you have broccoli on day one, you may not have it again until day five, but on day three you may have one of its relatives—such as Brussels sprouts.

Other food families include the legume family of peas, beans, dried beans, lentils, and pea pods. The citrus family includes oranges, grapefruit, tangerines, lemons, and limes. Apples and pears are related. Beef and veal are from the same animal source and so can only be eaten once in four days on a rotary diet. The same goes for pork and ham. But chicken and turkey are of two different species, and fish are generally quite unrelated to each other, so you can plan a wide variety of meals with these.

Grains must be assigned with their source in mind as well. Bran is the outer part of wheat, so you could choose to add either bran or wheat once in four days on this regimen. Grits are made of corn, therefore limiting your choice to one or the other within four days.

Many of the plants we eat belong to the same food families. Fortunately they do not generally represent the major allergens that create menu problems. Dairy products and grains which are part of the staple diet cause the most difficulty when it is necessary to eliminate one or both from the diet. The rotary diet makes it possible to identify which of these is giving trouble and which is not. With luck, the prescription may be to use the four-day rotary diet for only a few weeks—just long enough to pinpoint the food culprits.

Your doctor will supply you with a complete list of food families. Remember, the rotary diet should only be administered under the guidance of your doctor. The following guidelines, however, will help you to understand, plan, and cook a prescribed rotary diet.

ROTARY DIET MENU PLANNING

As you can see, planning a menu for such a four-day diversified diet can be quite complicated, or at least tedious, especially considering that you must also take balanced nutrition and already-known sensitivities into account. It's very important to keep the food interesting, though it should be cooked simply (broil, steam, or poach, and avoid sauces or other embellishments that could obscure ingredients). Meals should be planned with color and texture in mind, so the allergic person does not have to face a dish of bland, mushy food. It's bad enough to be restricted to this extent without having your palate bored and your senses dulled.

The easiest way to get started is to follow the four-day diversified rotary diet shown below. All the menus are patterned as described above, placing food relatives two days apart and otherwise calling for a food only once every four days. You can readily eliminate any food that has already been found to be an allergen and replace it with a food of similar nutritional value that seems to be safe.

While you can create your own rotary diet, this one can spare you a great deal of agonizing over food choices by providing a program that is palatable and also contributes to good health. Do discuss the possibility of vitamin and mineral supplementation with the prescribing physician, if this diet is advised for more than a few weeks.

Note that you may choose to serve portions of any size. This sample diet features a wide variety of food selections in order to maintain a good balance of nutrients and to avoid repetitions.

FOUR-DAY DIVERSIFIED ROTARY DIET

Day 1

Breakfast
Sliced orange or orange juice
Rye flatbread (no wheat)
Peanut butter

Lunch
Fillet of sole, flounder, or codfish
Carrots
Celery
Sliced pineapple

Dinner
Cooked artichoke or canned artichoke hearts
Broiled lamb chop or sliced lamb roast
Acorn squash, hubbard squash, mashed pumpkin,
   or a portion of melon
Spinach
Apricots

Day 2

Breakfast
Blueberries
2 eggs, boiled, poached, or scrambled in safflower oil

Lunch
Canned salmon or tuna, packed in water
Lettuce
Broiled or sliced tomato
Banana

Dinner
Broiled chicken or roast duck
Baked potato
Broccoli, Brussels sprouts, or cauliflower
Pear halves

Day 3

Breakfast
½ grapefruit
Cottage cheese, yogurt, or other cheese or milk product

Lunch
Shrimp, clams, lobster, mussels, scallops, or haddock
Rice
Peas, green beans, lima beans, or chickpeas
Sliced peaches, plums, or nectarines

Dinner
Beef or veal patties, or cooked, sliced beef or veal
Onions and mushrooms (may be sautéed in corn oil)
Zucchini or crookneck yellow squash
Corn
Strawberries

Day 4

Breakfast
    Cranberry juice
    Oatmeal cereal (no milk), pure wheat cereal, or
        wheat toast

Lunch
    Sliced turkey with natural gravy
    Asparagus
    Beets
    Figs

Dinner
    Pork chops, pork roast, baked bass or red snapper
    Baked sweet potato
    Cooked red or white cabbage *(see note below)*
    Baked apple or applesauce

NOTE: Broccoli, Brussels sprouts, or cauliflower may be substituted for cooked cabbage. Do not eat the exact same food again for four days, but you may eat another member of the cabbage family in two days.

If this diet seems prohibitive to your family, keep in mind that it can easily be expanded for the nonallergic people in your household. For instance, the allergic individual may be assigned only one grain in one meal during the four days, but the rest of the family may fill in with whatever grain products they desire. Also be sure you are aware of exactly what limitations this diet does *not* impose. If the allergic person is going to eat wheat pancakes made with eggs and milk, he or she may as well have butter on them and serve a glass of milk with it too, because amounts don't matter. Since those foods will be tabu for the next four days, why not have your fill of them now? You will have to cross wheat, eggs, and all dairy products off your list for four days.

Following this plan, if the patient chooses to have milk or a milk product, serve cheese, yogurt, or even a combination of several at the same meal, then it's off the list for four days. If, however, as a result of observing reactions while on the rotary diet, it is discovered that the allergic person can tolerate a small amount of milk or dairy products—called a low threshold of tolerance—then you would not want to load up on this substance because a higher amount would trigger the usual reaction. During the rotary diet, physical or behavioral reactions from each meal are noted, and the foods at a reaction-triggering meal would be served one at a time to track down the offending items.

You may find fruits and vegetables on this menu that you (or the allergic person) have never eaten before. Get into the spirit of adventure and give them a taste. Food habits can be very restricting, and there already are enough restrictions placed on the food sensitive person. One way out is to expand your taste horizons. Here are a few tips for adding variety to your meals on a rotary diet:

- If orange juice is suggested, an orange will do in its place. Certain types of fish are suggested, but you may vary your menu with others that you prefer.
- Learn the art of doubling up on a food item at one meal. For instance, if you serve corn on the cob, you may serve a pure cornmeal muffin with it. If you serve pasta (if there is no gluten allergy), you may serve wheat bread at the same meal.
- Another trick is to serve a juice and then also serve the fruit in whole form for a dessert. An example would be to start with apple juice and then serve applesauce for dessert.
- If the allergic person craves a piece of cake, save the wheat and eggs for that meal. Then serve an omelet and wheat toast too, or a similar combination, so that the eggs and wheat are repeated in one meal and then not eaten for four days.
- It's true that beef and veal are related, as are pork and ham, but lamb, goat, chicken, duck, turkey, and every other kind of poultry, fish, and meat stand alone. That gives you a wide variety of protein from which to choose.

- Vary your cooking oils by using safflower oil, olive oil, peanut oil, and every other salad oil that you can find. If you serve corn, then you may use corn oil for cooking at the same meal.
- Try not to combine a lot of vegetables in one salad. This will waste your choices for the four days. Instead, combine lettuce with just one vegetable or use one type of vegetable at each meal that lends itself to being sliced thin and marinated in vinegar and oil or water—such as thinly sliced cucumber or cooked beets served cold.

It is preferable not to have snacks, but when it is desired, be sure to choose a fruit or vegetable that has not been eaten in the four day period. This is the time when an unusual fruit selection, such as mango, papaya, blueberries, or cherries, would be a wise choice.

Now you can see why menus must be written down if you have to keep track of everything the allergic person eats within a period of four days. If you are cooking for an allergic person who is old enough to write, put a notebook in the kitchen and turn over the responsibility of recording any extras that may be eaten when you are away. A team effort may make this four-day rotary diet prescription a perfectly reasonable and delicious goal.

Once you have used this method to detect any reactions to food, the allergic person should be able to return to a normal way of eating and just eliminate the offending foods that were discovered. This can usually be done within a few weeks time, making it possible to repeat some meals that seem to have given a reaction to see whether it happens again. That meal, when broken apart and the foods served separately, should be an effective way of determining which foods to avoid.

Although the four-day rotary diet in this chapter has been designed to be as nutritious as possible, it should not be used as a role model for permanent balanced nutrition without medically prescribed vitamin and mineral supplementation. Do discuss all of these factors with your doctor for the best of health and the best of results.

4
The
Dairy-Free
Diet

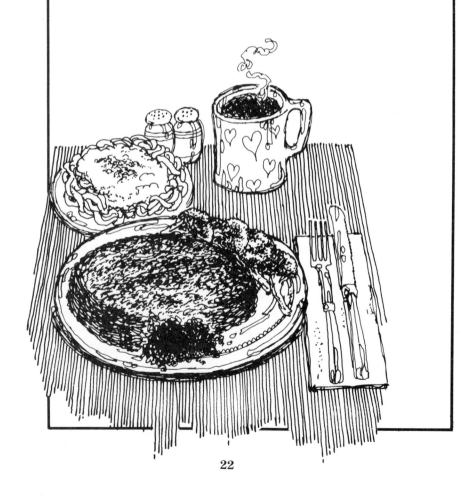

Sensitivity to dairy products is not unusual. Many people of non-European heredity do not have the lactase enzyme that is necessary for the digestion of cow's milk and therefore run into physical difficulties when products from this source are eaten. Others seem to have a sensitivity that manifests itself in emotional reactions, such as mood swings, or in skin eruptions, such as hives and rashes.

When dairy products have been pinpointed as the source of the difficulty they must be eliminated completely from the diet unless the allergic person is lacking the lactase enzyme but responds well to a new product that adds that enzyme to milk and makes it digestible. Also, some people cannot digest milk itself but can tolerate some dairy products that are manufactured through enzymatic reactions, such as yogurt and cheese. However, this chapter is intended for those who cannot have any dairy products at all. Before presenting recipes that will help those individuals learn how to eat well despite the restriction, we will examine eating habits in order to help them ferret out possible hidden sources of this food.

Those who are sensitive to all dairy products must eliminate milk, buttermilk, chocolate milk, skim milk, cream, sour cream, yogurt, ice cream, cheese, butter, and dried milk. Watch out for nondairy products that may have milk protein solids in the base. Label reading is a must.

When trying to determine the origin of foods by reading the labels, avoid any product that has the word "casein" or "caseinate" in it—this is a milk protein found in some "nondairy" substitutes and many other products. Also avoid any product that has an ingredient that begins with the letters "lact"— such as "lactose" or "lactic acid" as these too have a milk origin, and may cause problems for those sensitive to dairy products.

Avoid all bakery products, cocoa mixes, creamed soups, creamed sauces, and sherbets unless you are assured that they contain no milk-source product. Bake with pure white vegetable shortening. Read all margarine labels—some have milk protein solids added.

When dining out, the dairy-sensitive person should not order any creamed dishes, buttered vegetables, bread, cake, pies, puddings, junkets, omelets (unless it is specified that milk not be added to the eggs during preparation), rarebits, pancakes, quiche, custards, dishes with white or cream sauce, or waffles. It is highly likely that all these foods have been prepared with milk or butter. When in doubt, ask.

Your doctor may prescribe a soy milk formula substitute for a child's beverage, to replace cow's milk. Or it may be possible to obtain goat's milk, which may be satisfactory. Otherwise, it may be preferable to serve an allowable fruit juice. Combine it with club soda and you'll have a delicious bubbly beverage.

When you have to eliminate dairy products from the diet you are dispensing with our most important source of calcium. Calcium is important for the formation and continued good health of teeth and bones. It is therefore necessary to add some other high-calcium foods to the diet every day. These include dark green leafy vegetables, canned salmon and sardines (with the bones mashed in), and goat's cheese (if there is no sensitivity to it). Also, discuss calcium supplementation with your doctor. Do not use a health food store manager to prescribe the kind of calcium that is best for you, unless you are dealing with a trained clinical nutritionist—self-medication of minerals may be well intentioned but may also involve the wrong selection for your particular needs.

When trying to bake without milk, it is sometimes possible to substitute a compatible fruit juice, particularly if the recipe requires a small amount; such as ¼ cup. Otherwise it is possible to use plain water as the liquid. Do not attempt to do this if you are supposed to use more than ½ cup of milk, because the end result may be a waste of ingredients and time.

It's better to find recipes, such as those in this chapter, that have been devised without any dairy products. You can make substitutions for butter by using shortening or a margarine with no milk solids and salvage some of your favorite recipes that way. Notice that some of the following recipes are free of more than dairy products. If someone in your home has such multiple allergies, you will rejoice in the multiple-allergy recipe chapter, which eliminates all three of the major causes of sensitivity—dairy products, eggs, and gluten flours. Even if dairy products are the only problem, you will find additional dairy-free recipes in Chapter 7, which contains multiple-allergy recipes.

APPETIZERS

Egg–Peanut Butter Spread

DAIRY-FREE
GLUTEN-FREE

Here's a high-protein spread with a punch of raw vegetables for good measure. If there is no gluten sensitivity, wheat, oat, and rye flour crackers may be used.

4 hard-cooked eggs, shells removed
¼ cup shredded carrots
¼ cup finely chopped celery
3 tablespoons mayonnaise
2 tablespoons soft smooth peanut butter

Chop eggs coarsely. Add carrots and celery. Combine mayonnaise and peanut butter until smooth; add to egg mixture and mix well. Serve as a spread on rice crackers or mounded on greens as a salad.

Makes about 1½ cups

Tuna Chutney Spread

DAIRY-FREE

Chutney may be found among the relishes in your supermarket. It gives an unusual tang to tuna.

1 7-ounce can waterpack tuna, drained
4 tablespoons chutney
2 tablespoons mayonnaise
1 tablespoon chopped olives
Dairy-free crackers

Mash tuna. Mix with chutney, mayonnaise, and olives. Chill until ready to use. Spread on dairy-free crackers or on sliced cucumbers.

Makes 1 cup

Bacon Date Rolls

DAIRY-FREE
GLUTEN-FREE

Here's a delicious mouthful that can be prepared ahead of time and broiled at the last minute. If desired, egg white may be omitted.

12 slices lean bacon
36 pitted dates
1 egg white, beaten slightly
¼ cup soft brown sugar

Cut bacon slices into thirds. Wrap each piece around a pitted date. Dip in beaten egg white. Roll in brown sugar. Place on a broiling pan. Broil for 6 minutes or until bacon is crisp. Serve hot.

Makes 3 dozen appetizers

Sardine Patties

DAIRY-FREE

The dough from this recipe may be stuffed with any other dairy-free mixture, such as tuna and crushed pineapple, or chopped mushrooms and soy sauce. Dough may also be folded over into a half-moon shape, if preferred.

1 cup flour
½ cup vegetable shortening
1 teaspoon baking powder
½ teaspoon salt
2 4½-ounce cans boneless sardines, drained
1 tablespoon lemon juice
2 tablespoons finely chopped onion
1 egg, beaten

Combine flour, shortening, baking powder, and salt into a dough. Roll out ¼-inch thick and cut into rounds with the rim of a 4-inch drinking glass. Mash sardines fine; mix with lemon juice and onion. Place 1 teaspoon of mixture into the center of each round of dough. Gather edges up to form a frill. Prick top with a fork in several places. Brush top surfaces with beaten egg. Bake in a 350°F. oven for 30 minutes, or until lightly browned. Serve hot.

Makes about 2 dozen appetizers

Chopped Herring

DAIRY-FREE
GLUTEN-FREE

When the dairy-sensitive must pass up the cheese tray, have a few spreads such as this available. Hard-cooked egg may be omitted, if desired.

1 12-ounce jar herring in white sauce, drained
1 hard-cooked egg
½ apple, cored and peeled
1 small onion, diced fine
¼ teaspoon pepper
½ teaspoon sugar

Empty herring into a chopping bowl. Add hard-cooked egg, apple, onion, pepper, and sugar. Chop very fine. Serve as a spread with dairy-free crackers or cucumber slices.

Makes 1 cup

Spicy Deviled Eggs

DAIRY-FREE
GLUTEN-FREE

It's so nice to provide a tasty mouthful for those who must skip the sour cream dips. Here's a way to make a zesty egg offering.

6 hard-cooked eggs, shelled
1 tablespoon stuffed olives, finely chopped
2 tablespoons mayonnaise
1 teaspoon prepared mustard
⅛ teaspoon pepper
Paprika
Parsley

Split eggs in half lengthwise. Scoop egg yolks carefully out of their sockets and place in a bowl. Mash together. Add olives, mayonnaise, mustard, and pepper. Refill the egg white sockets with this mixture. Swirl the tops decoratively. Sprinkle with paprika and garnish with bits of parsley. Chill until ready to serve.

Makes 1 dozen

Stuffed Mushrooms

DAIRY-FREE
EGG-FREE

These may be broiled ahead of time and reheated just before serving. Cornstarch may be used in place of flour if necessary.

24 mushrooms, 1-inch diameter
1 teaspoon flour
2 tablespoons chopped onion
1 tablespoon finely chopped parsley
¼ teaspoon oregano
¼ teaspoon salt
⅛ teaspoon pepper
2 tablespoons dairy-free margarine

Wash mushrooms and remove stems. Trim ends of stems and chop very fine. Add flour, onion, parsley, oregano, salt, and pepper to chopped stems; stuff mixture into mushroom cavities. Dot each with a bit of margarine. Broil for 6 minutes, or until mushrooms are hot and lightly browned on top.

Makes 2 dozen appetizers

SOUPS

Mushroom Barley Soup

DAIRY-FREE
EGG-FREE

Remember that barley is one of the gluten grains, so if there is a sensitivity to wheat and other glutens, this soup can still be made by substituting ½ cup rice for the barley and simmering with the soup meat ½ hour instead of an hour.

1 cup barley
1 pound soup meat or several beef bones
2 quarts water
1 onion, diced
2 carrots, scraped and diced
2 stalks celery, diced fine
½ pound fresh mushrooms, sliced
1 teaspoon salt
¼ teaspoon pepper
1 sprig fresh dillweed or 1 teaspoon dried dillweed

Simmer barley and soup meat in 2 quarts of water for 1 hour. Skim surface with a large spoon to remove residue. Add the remaining ingredients and simmer, stirring occasionally, for another hour.

Makes 8 servings

Cream of Carrot Soup

DAIRY-FREE
EGG-FREE

This recipe shows how to thicken a soup without using dairy products. To avoid lumps, be sure to stir liquid gradually into the thickened roux. If there is a gluten allergy, substitute cornstarch or arrowroot powder for the wheat flour.

2 pounds carrots, scraped
  and sliced
1 cup water
1 teaspoon sugar
½ teaspoon salt
¼ teaspoon pepper

1 medium onion, chopped
2 tablespoons dairy-free
  margarine
2 tablespoons flour
1 cup chicken broth

Cook carrots, water, sugar, salt, and pepper together until carrots are soft enough to mash. Puree in food processor or blender. Sauté onion in margarine. Stir in flour and stir until thick. Gradually add chicken broth, stirring and cooking until thickened. Add carrots and carrot liquid. Cook five minutes, stirring occasionally.

Makes 4 servings

Potato Leek Soup

DAIRY-FREE
EGG-FREE

Try to buy large thick leeks for the best flavor. Cornstarch or arrowroot powder may be substituted for wheat flour, if necessary.

4 large potatoes, peeled and
  diced
2 large leeks, sliced thin
  (including tops)
2 stalks celery, diced fine
1 sprig dillweed
3 cups water

1 teaspoon salt
¼ teaspoon pepper
2 tablespoons dairy-free
  margarine
2 tablespoons flour
1 cup Chicken Broth
  (see recipe)

Place potatoes, leeks, celery, dillweed, water, salt, and pepper in a large saucepan. Simmer for 20 minutes, or until potatoes are very tender. Mash potatoes into their liquid. In a separate saucepan, melt margarine and stir in flour. Cook until thickened, stirring constantly. Gradually add chicken broth and stir until all is thick and smooth. Gradually add this mixture to the potato soup, stirring constantly. Cook for several minutes and serve hot.

Makes 4 servings

Lemon Rice Soup

GLUTEN-FREE
DAIRY-FREE

This Greek soup is dainty in appearance and lovely to sip. Keep the heat low as you add the egg—you're not making egg-drop soup today!

1 quart Chicken Broth (see recipe)
3 tablespoons raw rice
½ teaspoon salt
¼ teaspoon dried dillweed
2 eggs
3 tablespoons lemon juice
4 thin slices lemon
Paprika

Place broth, rice, salt, and dillweed in a saucepan. Cover and cook for 15 minutes, or until rice is tender. Beat eggs until fluffy and lemon-colored; add lemon juice. Slowly stir egg mixture into the soup as it simmers. Remove from heat and serve at once. Add a thin slice of lemon with a dash of paprika to garnish each bowl of soup.

Makes 4 servings

Creamy Tomato Soup

DAIRY-FREE

Soy milk has a flavor of its own, but here it is nicely disguised and helpful to cream a dairy-free soup. Float some freshly popped corn on top, if the spirit moves you.

3 cups tomato juice
⅓ cup dried soy milk
1 tablespoon dairy-free margarine
1 tablespoon lemon juice

1 teaspoon sugar
½ teaspoon salt
½ teaspoon dried basil
⅛ teaspoon pepper
¼ cup pastina

Combine all ingredients except pastina in a saucepan. Stir until smooth while cooking over low heat. When margarine has melted, add pastina and cook 5 minutes.

Makes 4 servings

Tomato Clam Soup

DAIRY-FREE
EGG-FREE

This soup may be served in clear form, if desired, by omitting the roux of margarine and flour. Cornstarch or arrowroot powder may be used in place of wheat flour, when indicated.

3 cups tomato juice
1 cup clam juice
1 teaspoon lemon juice
¼ teaspoon salt
⅛ teaspoon pepper
¼ teaspoon oregano
1 tablespoon dairy-free margarine
1 tablespoon flour
½ cup Chicken Broth (see recipe)

Combine tomato juice, clam juice, lemon juice, salt, pepper, and oregano in a large saucepan. Heat through. In a small saucepan, melt margarine and stir in flour until thick; gradually stir in chicken broth. When thickened, gradually stir into tomato/clam juice mixture. Cook and stir for several minutes before serving.

Makes 4 servings

Creamy Pumpkin Soup

DAIRY-FREE
EGG-FREE

Pumpkin lends itself so nicely to a thick winter soup. Thicken with cornstarch or arrowroot powder in place of wheat flour if there is a gluten allergy.

¼ cup finely chopped onion
4 tablespoons dairy-free margarine
2 tablespoons flour
1 cup chicken broth
1 cup cooked canned pumpkin
½ teaspoon ground nutmeg
½ teaspoon sugar
¼ teaspoon salt
⅛ teaspoon pepper
1 cup water

Sauté onion in 2 tablespoons of margarine. Add remaining margarine and flour. Gradually add chicken broth, stirring constantly until mixture is thickened. Stir in pumpkin, nutmeg, sugar, salt, and pepper. Gradually stir in water. Heat, stirring occasionally.

Makes 4 servings

ENTREES

Beef

Oatmeal Meatloaf

DAIRY-FREE

Those who have a gluten allergy may substitute uncooked rice cereal for the oats. Either way, it is a very tasty meatloaf.

1½ pounds ground beef
¾ cup uncooked oat cereal
1 egg, beaten
1 cup tomato juice
1 small onion, grated

¾ teaspoon salt
¼ teaspoon pepper
1 tablespoon minced
 fresh parsley

Combine all ingredients and mix well. Pack into a loaf pan and bake in a 350°F. oven for 1 hour.

Makes 6 servings

Fluffy Meatloaf

DAIRY-FREE

Grated potato is the secret of a fluffy meatloaf. Add extra minced onion if you like the flavor.

2 pounds ground beef
2 eggs
2 slices dairy-free bread (see note)
½ cup cold water
1 small potato, peeled and grated
¼ cup chopped parsley
2 tablespoons minced onion
1 teaspoon salt
¼ teaspoon pepper

Combine ground beef and eggs. Soak bread in water and shred into meat. Add grated potatoes, parsley, onion, salt, and pepper. Turn into a 9-by-5-inch loaf pan or form into a loaf shape in a shallow baking pan. Bake in a preheated 350°F. oven for 1 hour.

Makes 8 servings

NOTE: For the bread in this recipe, use White Bread or Egg-Free Whole Wheat Bread (see recipes), with the dairy-free margarine substitute, or choose another dairy-free bread from this book (see index).

Orange Meatloaf

DAIRY-FREE

Here is a meatloaf that has a delectable aroma. Bake it in muffin tins for individual servings and freeze the extras.

1½ pounds lean ground beef
1 cup cooked mashed carrots
1 egg, lightly beaten
½ cup orange juice
½ cup dairy-free breadcrumbs (see note on p. 35)
½ cup chopped onion
¼ cup chopped parsley
½ teaspoon salt
2 tablespoons orange marmalade

Combine all ingredients except the marmalade; mix well. Pack into an 8½-by-4½-inch loaf pan or into muffin tins. Spread marmalade thinly over the top of the meatloaf. Bake loaf in a 350° F. oven for 1 hour, or muffins for 40 minutes.

Makes 6 servings

Swedish Meatballs

DAIRY-FREE
GLUTEN-FREE

Note the nutmeg and ginger that give the zest of Scandinavian flavor. These make an excellent hors d'oeuvre. Combine apricot jam and a bit of mustard for a zippy dip.

1 pound ground beef
½ pound ground veal
1 egg
1 cup hot mashed potatoes
2 tablespoons grated onion
½ teaspoon salt
⅛ teaspoon pepper
¼ teaspoon nutmeg
⅛ teaspoon ginger
2 tablespoons oil
¼ cup water

Combine all ingredients except oil and water; form into 1-inch balls. Heat oil in a large skillet; brown meatballs over low heat, shaking pan occasionally to brown all sides. Add ¼ cup water, cover, and simmer 20 minutes.

Makes about 4 dozen meatballs

Curried Meatballs

DAIRY-FREE

To make this recipe gluten-free, substitute cornstarch for flour and replace the breadcrumbs with ¹/₂ cup uncooked cream of rice cereal.

2 pounds ground beef
1 onion, chopped fine
1¼ cups fine dairy-free breadcrumbs (see note on p. 35)
2 eggs
¾ teaspoon curry powder
½ teaspoon salt
¼ teaspoon pepper
2 cloves garlic, diced
1 cup flour
2 tablespoons olive oil
1 cup water
2 8-ounce cans tomato sauce
¼ teaspoon oregano

Combine beef, onion, and breadcrumbs in a bowl. Add eggs, curry powder, salt, and pepper. Add half the diced garlic. Form mixture into 1½-inch balls. Roll each ball lightly in flour. Heat oil and remaining garlic in a large skillet; brown meatballs on all sides, then remove and set aside. Pour off oil/fat from pan. Add water, tomato sauce and oregano to the skillet. Mix the remaining flour with enough water to form a thin paste and stir into the tomato mixture. Add the meatballs; cover and simmer about 25 minutes.

Makes 8 servings

Beef Noodle Skillet

DAIRY-FREE

Those with a gluten and/or egg sensitivity can serve this dish on hot cooked brown rice with equal pleasure.

1 8-ounce can tomato sauce
½ cup water
1 teaspoon salt
¼ teaspoon pepper
1 teaspoon oregano
¼ teaspoon thyme
1 teaspoon Worcestershire sauce
3 tablespoons cooking oil
1 pound lean ground beef
1 cup chopped onions
1 clove garlic, minced
1 green pepper, diced
2 cups sliced celery
½ cup chopped parsley
8 ounces wide egg noodles, cooked and drained

Combine tomato sauce, water, salt, pepper, oregano, thyme, and Worcestershire sauce; set aside. Heat oil in a large skillet; add beef and stir constantly until browned. Remove meat with a slotted spoon and set aside. Add onions, garlic, green pepper, celery, and parsley to skillet; sauté until tender. Return meat, tomato sauce mixture, and hot cooked noodles to skillet; toss lightly and heat through.

Makes 4 servings

Roast Sirloin of Beef

DAIRY-FREE
EGG-FREE

Cornstarch may be used in place of flour to make this gluten-free, or both may be omitted.

2 tablespoons flour
½ teaspoon salt
½ teaspoon powdered onion

½ teaspoon paprika
1 beef sirloin roast,
    about 4 pounds

Combine flour, salt, onion powder, and paprika; pat mixture all over surface of roast. Place on a rack in a shallow roasting pan. Place in a preheated 350°F. oven and roast for about 20 minutes to the pound for rare, 25 minutes per pound for medium, and 30 minutes per pound for well done. Transfer roast to platter to rest before carving. For a quick pan gravy, pour a cup of boiling water into the pan of drippings; scrape and stir. Then heat on top of the range. Strain before serving, if preferred.

Makes 8 servings

Sauerbraten

DAIRY-FREE
EGG-FREE

The secret of sauerbraten lies in marinating the flavor into the meat for several days before cooking. Cornstarch may be used instead of flour for the gluten-sensitive.

2 cups white vinegar
1 cup water
1 tablespoon brown sugar
1 teaspoon ground ginger
2 bay leaves
6 whole peppercorns

2 onions, sliced
1 beef round or brisket
    roast, about 4 pounds
½ cup flour
¼ cup oil

Combine vinegar, water, sugar, ginger, bay leaves, pepper-corns, and onions in a saucepan. Heat for 10 minutes, then cool. Place meat in a large deep bowl and cover with the cooled marinade. Refrigerate for 2 days, turning meat morning and night. Remove meat from marinade and wipe dry. Pat with flour. Heat oil and brown meat in it on all sides. Place meat in a Dutch oven and add 1 cup of the marinade. Simmer, covered, until meat is tender. Remove and slice. Serve with gravy.

Makes 8 servings

Swiss Steak

DAIRY-FREE
EGG-FREE

Here grapefruit juice is used as both a liquid and a tenderizer. Use cornstarch instead of flour to eliminate gluten.

1 slice top round beef steak, about 2 pounds
½ teaspoon salt
¼ teaspoon pepper
¼ teaspoon paprika
2 tablespoons flour
3 tablespoons oil
1 onion, sliced
1 cup grapefruit juice

Wipe beef slice dry. Combine salt, pepper, paprika, and flour; pound mixture into surface of the steak on all sides. Heat oil in a Dutch oven; add onion and cook until golden. Add steak and brown on all sides. Pour grapefruit juice around steak; cover and simmer for 1 hour, or until tender.

Makes 6 servings

Veal

Stuffed Breast of Veal

DAIRY-FREE

Sprinkle additional rosemary over the top of the veal roast if you like the flavor. The egg may be replaced by ⅓ cup of apple juice.

1 large breast of veal, about 4 pounds
2 onions, diced
2 tablespoons oil
2 cups coarse dairy-free breadcrumbs (see note on p. 35)
2 apples, diced
½ teaspoon salt
¼ teaspoon pepper
½ teaspoon rosemary
1 egg, beaten
½ teaspoon paprika

Cut a pocket in the breast of veal for stuffing. Sauté onions in oil in a skillet until onions are golden. Remove from heat and stir in breadcrumbs, apples, salt, pepper, and rosemary. Add beaten egg and mix well. Fill cavity of the veal pocket with this mixture. Place roast in an open pan and sprinkle with paprika. Roast at 325°F. until well done (about 30 minutes per pound of meat), basting often with pan drippings.

Makes 6 servings

Veal Banana Loaf

DAIRY-FREE

Oats contain gluten. Uncooked cream of rice cereal may be substituted for oats in this recipe. Those who are sensitive to beef should not eat veal. Lamb may be substituted with fine results.

1½ pounds ground veal
1 cup mashed ripe bananas
½ cup uncooked quick oats
1 egg
1 onion, chopped fine
2 tablespoons chopped parsley
½ teaspoon salt
¼ teaspoon dried thyme
¼ teaspoon white pepper

Combine veal, bananas, oats, and egg until well blended. Add onion, parsley, salt, thyme, and pepper. Pack into an 8-by-4-inch loaf pan. Bake in a 350°F. oven for 1 hour.

Makes 6 servings

Pork

Breaded Pork Chops

DAIRY-FREE

Those with a pork allergy may use veal or lamb chops in this recipe. Be sure the breadcrumbs are dairy-free or use matzo meal instead.

6 rib pork chops, cut 1-inch thick
1 egg, lightly beaten
¼ teaspoon dry mustard
½ cup dairy-free breadcrumbs (see note on p. 35)
½ teaspoon salt
3 tablespoons olive oil
½ cup water
1 onion, sliced
1 apple, peeled and sliced

Dip pork chops first into egg beaten with mustard and then into combined breadcrumbs and salt, coating well. Heat oil in a skillet; brown chops on all sides. Place browned chops in a baking dish; pour water around the chops and add onion slices and apple slices. Cover tightly with a lid or aluminum foil. Bake in a 350°F. oven for 1 hour, or until tender.

Makes 6 servings

Sweet and Sour Pork Chops

DAIRY-FREE
EGG-FREE

Remember to cook pork until well done for safest results. Chops may be dusted with a gluten-free flour, if desired.

2 tablespoons flour
1 teaspoon paprika
6 pork chops
6 whole cloves

2 tablespoons cooking oil
1 tablespoon brown sugar
½ cup orange juice
¼ teaspoon ginger

Combine flour and paprika; dust chops lightly with the mixture. Insert a whole clove in the center of each pork chop. Heat oil in a large skillet; brown chops on both sides over medium heat. Stir brown sugar into orange juice; add ginger. Pour over chops. Cover and simmer over low heat for 30 minutes, or until fork tender.

Makes 6 servings

Fried Pork Chops and Apples

DAIRY-FREE
EGG-FREE

Apples have a natural affinity for pork chops. Here they are flavored with the drippings from the frying chops. Delectable!

6 well-trimmed pork chops
2 tablespoons flour
¼ teaspoon powdered sage
¼ teaspoon salt
⅛ teaspoon pepper
¼ cup cooking oil
2 apples

Dip pork chops in a combination of flour, sage, salt, and pepper; coat lightly. Heat oil in a skillet. Brown chops on both sides and cook for 30 minutes, until fork tender. Remove chops to a warm platter. Cut apples across the core in ½-inch slices; cut out core in each slice. Fry the apple slices in the same skillet, adding a little more oil, if needed. Turn apple slices when they are browned. Serve with the pork chops.

Makes 6 servings

Lamb

Lamb Loaf

DAIRY-FREE

Use leanest ground lamb for this loaf, preferably from the shoulder or leg. Serve with mint jelly.

1½ pounds ground lamb
1 small onion, grated
1 chopped green pepper
1 large tomato
1 egg, slightly beaten
¼ cup dairy-free breadcrumbs
¼ teaspoon crushed rosemary
¼ teaspoon salt
⅛ teaspoon pepper

Combine ground lamb, onion, and green pepper. Cut up tomato and puree in an electric blender or food processor; add to lamb mixture. Add beaten egg, breadcrumbs, rosemary, salt, and pepper. Mix well. Place mixture in a 9-by-5-inch loaf pan. Bake for 1 hour.

Makes 6 servings

Curried Lamb in Applesauce

DAIRY-FREE
EGG-FREE

When you'd like to dress up leftover lamb roast, cut it into cubes and serve it curried over rice. Substitute cornstarch for flour, if necessary.

2 cups applesauce
2 teaspoons curry powder
½ teaspoon rosemary
2 tablespoons flour

2 cups beef bouillon
6 cups cubed cooked lamb
4 cups cooked rice

Combine applesauce, curry powder, rosemary, and flour. Gradually stir in bouillon. Cook, stirring constantly, until thickened. Add lamb cubes and heat through. Mound hot rice on a platter and spoon curried lamb over the rice.

Makes 8 servings

Poultry*

Stuffed Roast Chicken

DAIRY-FREE

Cooked rice may be substituted for the breadcrumbs. Either way, don't pack the stuffing or you may cause the breast to burst.

1 roasting chicken, 4–5 pounds
1 teaspoon salt
2 cups soft dairy-free breadcrumbs (see note on p. 35)
2 tablespoons chopped parsley
2 tablespoons chopped celery leaves
2 tablespoons chopped onion
¼ teaspoon thyme
¼ cup water
¼ teaspoon paprika

Wash chicken and pat dry. Sprinkle with salt inside and out. Combine breadcrumbs, parsley, celery leaves, onion, and thyme. Add water. Spoon stuffing into chicken cavity, being careful not to pack it too tightly. Sprinkle paprika over chicken. Place chicken on a rack in a roasting pan and roast in a preheated 325° F. oven for about 2½ hours, or until tender.

Makes 6 servings

---

*Additional dairy-free poultry recipes can be found in chapters 5, 6, and 7 (see index).

Chicken Marengo

DAIRY-FREE
EGG-FREE

Black olives give this dish its unique tang. Use cornstarch in place of flour to make this gluten-free.

2 broiler chickens, cut up
¼ cup flour
1 teaspoon paprika
¼ teaspoon black pepper
¼ cup oil
1 green pepper, diced

2 tomatoes, peeled and
  quartered
½ cup sliced ripe olives
1 teaspoon oregano
1 teaspoon salt
1 cup chicken broth

Wash and dry chicken parts. Combine flour, paprika, and black pepper. Heat oil in a skillet. Dredge chicken parts in flour mixture; brown in oil. Transfer to a baking dish. Add tomatoes, green pepper, olives, oregano, and salt. Combine chicken broth with 1 tablespoon of remaining flour mixture and pour into skillet to cook and thicken, stirring constantly. Pour over chicken in baking dish. Cover tightly and bake in a 350° F. oven for 35 minutes, or until tender.

Makes 8 servings

Chicken Cacciatore

DAIRY-FREE
EGG-FREE

This will be gluten-free if you use cornstarch in place of the flour. Serve on rice or noodles, as your allergy dictates.

2 broiler chickens, cut up
½ cup flour
1 teaspoon salt
½ teaspoon paprika
¼ teaspoon garlic powder
⅛ teaspoon pepper
¼ cup olive oil

1 16-ounce can tomatoes in
  natural liquid
1 cup Chicken Broth
  (see recipe)
2 sweet Italian peppers,
  seeded and diced fine
½ pound fresh mushrooms

Dredge each chicken part in a mixture of flour, salt, paprika, garlic powder, and pepper. Heat oil in a Dutch oven; brown chicken on all sides. Add tomatoes, chicken broth, peppers, and sliced mushrooms. Cover and simmer over low heat for 1 hour, or until tender.

Makes 6–8 servings

Lemon Chicken

DAIRY-FREE
EGG-FREE

A tantalizing lemon marinade lifts this chicken into the realm of the sublime. Using cornstarch in place of flour will allow the gluten-sensitive to enjoy it too, but don't forget to check the soy sauce label for wheat products.

¼ **cup lemon juice**
¼ **cup water**
¼ **cup salad oil**
1 **tablespoon grated lemon rind**
1 **tablespoon pure soy sauce**
1 **clove garlic, minced**
1 **teaspoon salt**
¼ **teaspoon pepper**
1 **fryer chicken, cut up (about 3 pounds)**
¼ **cup flour**
1 **teaspoon paprika**

Mix together lemon juice, water, salad oil, lemon rind, soy sauce, garlic, salt, and pepper. Pour over chicken and refrigerate, covered, for several hours. When ready to cook, remove chicken from marinade and pat dry with paper towels. Dip into a mixture of flour and paprika, coating lightly. Arrange in one layer in a greased baking dish. Bake in a 400°F. oven for 30 minutes; turn chicken and pour remaining lemon juice marinade over the chicken. Bake for 30 minutes more, or until tender.

Makes 4 servings

Chicken Fricassee

DAIRY-FREE

The use of cornstarch in place of flour will make this recipe gluten-free. If desired, the egg may be eliminated from the meatballs.

**Wings, necks, backs, thighs, and legs of 2 chickens
    (about 3 pounds each)**
¼ **cup flour**
2 **onions, diced**
¼ **cup rendered chicken fat, or cooking oil**
1 **cup boiling chicken broth**
½ **pound lean ground beef**
1 **egg, beaten**
¼ **cup cold water**
¼ **teaspoon salt**
⅛ **teaspoon pepper**
1 **tablespoon chopped parsley**
¼ **cup cold water**

Dredge chicken parts in flour. Sauté onions in chicken fat in a deep saucepan. Add chicken parts and brown on all sides. Add chicken broth, cover, and simmer. Combine ground beef, beaten egg, ¼ cup cold water, salt, pepper, and chopped parsley. Form tiny meatballs and add to chicken. Cook for 20 minutes over very low heat. To thicken gravy, combine 2 tablespoons of flour with ¼ cup cold water; stir several tablespoons of the hot gravy into this mixture and then pour all back into the saucepan, stirring. Continue to stir until a boiling point is reached and the gravy thickens. Add additional salt and pepper to taste. Serve over rice, if desired.

Makes 6–8 servings

Fish

Halibut Salad

DAIRY-FREE
GLUTEN-FREE

This is a delicious way to use leftover cooked fish. Dillweed adds a subtle flavor.

1 pound halibut, cooked and flaked	¼ teaspoon salt
2 tablespoons lemon juice	¼ teaspoon dried dillweed
½ cup chopped celery	½ cup Mayonnaise (see recipe)

Mix flaked fish, lemon juice, celery, salt, and dillweed. Add mayonnaise and mix thoroughly.

Makes 2¹/₂ cups

Salmon Loaf

DAIRY-FREE

Here's an inexpensively delicious way to serve six people. Mashed potatoes may be substituted for breadcrumbs to make the loaf gluten-free.

1 16-ounce can salmon	¼ cup chopped scallions
½ cup soft fresh dairy-free breadcrumbs (see note p. 35)	½ teaspoon salt
	½ teaspoon celery salt
2 tablespoons chopped fresh parsley	⅛ teaspoon pepper
	1 egg, well beaten

Drain and flake salmon. Add crumbs, scallions, parsley, salt, celery salt, pepper, and beaten egg; mix well. Pat into a greased 8-by-4-inch loaf pan. Bake at 350°F. for 30 minutes.

Makes 6 servings

Clam Fritters

DAIRY-FREE

Cornstarch may be used in place of flour for the gluten-sensitive. For crispy fritters, be sure that the oil is hot—test by dropping a cube of bread into oil; it should turn brown and crispy immediately.

1 egg
¼ cup clam juice
½ cup wheat flour
2 teaspoons baking powder
½ teaspoon salt
⅛ teaspoon pepper
2 cups finely chopped raw clams
2 tablespoons grated onion
1 cup salad oil

Beat egg; add clam juice. Stir in flour, baking powder, salt, and pepper. Add chopped clams and onion. Heat oil in a skillet. Drop clam mixture by tablespoonfuls into hot oil; brown on one side, then turn and brown other side. Remove with a slotted spoon to drain on paper towels.

Makes 4 servings

Fried Scallops

DAIRY-FREE

Use uncooked cream of rice cereal for under and over coatings if there is a gluten allergy. Skip the mayonnaise for those who must eat egg-free.

1 pint fresh scallops, about 1 pound
½ cup flour
1 cup Mayonnaise (see recipe)
1 cup soda cracker crumbs
1 cup cooking oil

Cut large scallops in half; if using bay scallops, leave them whole. Roll in flour, dip in mayonnaise until evenly coated, then roll in crumbs. Pour oil into a skillet and heat until a 1-inch bread cube turns brown in 40 seconds. Fry scallops in hot oil until golden brown, about 3 minutes. Drain on paper towels.

Makes 4 servings

Salmon Croquettes

DAIRY-FREE

This mixture can be prepared in the morning and then shaped just before dinner. Chilling is a must to make the mixture easy to handle.

1 16-ounce can salmon, drained and flaked
½ cup soft dairy-free breadcrumbs (see note on p. 35)
½ cup Mayonnaise (see recipe)
2 eggs, beaten
2 tablespoons diced green pepper
1 tablespoon grated onion
½ teaspoon salt
¼ teaspoon paprika
¼ teaspoon dry mustard
1 teaspoon lemon juice
Additional soft dairy-free breadcrumbs
¼ cup cooking oil

Combine salmon, ½ cup breadcrumbs, mayonnaise, eggs, green pepper, onion, salt, paprika, mustard, and lemon juice. Chill mixture for two to three hours. Shape salmon mixture into 12 small or 8 large croquettes. Coat with the additional breadcrumbs until well covered. Heat oil in a large skillet over medium heat; brown croquettes on all sides. Drain on paper towels.

Makes 4 servings

EGGS

Fluffy Scrambled Eggs

DAIRY-FREE
GLUTEN-FREE

No, you don't have to add milk to make creamy eggs. Here it's done with a bit of mayonnaise instead.

4 eggs	2 tablespoons mayonnaise
¼ cup water	2 teaspoons chopped chives
¼ teaspoon salt	1 tablespoon dairy-free
⅛ teaspoon pepper	margarine

Beat eggs. Add water, salt, pepper, mayonnaise, and chopped chives. Melt margarine in a large skillet. Pour egg mixture into skillet and cook over medium heat, pushing solidified egg aside and allowing liquid egg to contact the skillet. Cook until eggs are set but still moist. Serve at once.

Makes 2 servings

Eggs à La Russe

DAIRY-FREE
GLUTEN-FREE

Use this as a first course, placing two egg halves on each plate. Garnish with sprigs of fresh parsley.

4 hard-cooked eggs, shelled	2 teaspoons capers
½ cup mayonnaise	Paprika
½ cup chili sauce	

Split hard-cooked eggs in half lengthwise. Stir mayonnaise and chili sauce together. Spoon over the eggs, letting some of the egg show. Garnish with capers. Sprinkle with a dash of paprika. Serve cold.

Makes 4 servings

Baked Egg in a Tomato

DAIRY-FREE
GLUTEN-FREE

Shred some ham into the tomato before breaking the egg, and you will have an extra punch of protein for breakfast.

1 large tomato	Dash of salt
1 egg	Dash of pepper
½ teaspoon chopped chives	

Scoop out some of the pulp from the top of the tomato. Place on a baking pan. Break egg carefully into the tomato. Sprinkle with chives, salt, and pepper. Bake in a 350°F. oven for about 15 minutes, or until egg reaches desired firmness. Serve at once.

Makes 1 serving

Eggs and Corn Tarragon

DAIRY-FREE
GLUTEN-FREE

Fresh corn is best, but if fresh is unavailable, drained canned niblet corn can be substituted in this recipe. Add diced green pepper, if desired.

2 ears of corn, cooked	2 tablespoons water
2 tablespoons dairy-free margarine	¼ teaspoon tarragon
	⅛ teaspoon salt
4 eggs	Dash of pepper

Cut corn from the cobs. Melt margarine in a large skillet; add corn and cook for 1 minute. Beat eggs, water, tarragon, salt, and pepper together and pour over corn. As the mixture cooks push it toward the center of the skillet to permit liquid mixture to run toward the edge. Serve as soon as eggs are set.

Makes 2 servings

Tomato Pepper Omelet

DAIRY-FREE
GLUTEN-FREE

In this version of an omelet, the filling is cooked into the egg. Add other compatible leftover cooked vegetables as desired.

2 tablespoons dairy-free margarine	1 tomato, peeled and diced
1 small onion, diced fine	2 tablespoons water
1 green pepper, seeded and diced	⅛ teaspoon salt
4 eggs	Dash pepper

Melt margarine in a skillet; add onion, green pepper, and tomato. Stir and cook for several minutes or until onion is translucent. Beat eggs and water together. Add salt and pepper. Pour egg mixture over vegetables in the skillet. Push mixture towards the center of the skillet as it solidifies, letting the liquid egg run to the edge. Fold over and serve.

Makes 2 servings

VEGETABLES AND VEGETABLE SAUCES*

Confetti Cole Slaw

DAIRY-FREE
GLUTEN-FREE

Here's a cole slaw that includes carrots and green pepper. A vegetable salad with creamy dressing!

1 cup Mayonnaise (see recipe)	⅛ teaspoon dry mustard
1 tablespoon vinegar	⅛ teaspoon tarragon
2 teaspoons sugar	2 cups shredded cabbage
1 tablespoon grated onion	1 green pepper, seeded and diced fine
¼ teaspoon salt	
⅛ teaspoon pepper	2 carrots, shredded

---

*You will find very few vegetable recipes here, as margarine can be used in place of butter on vegetables; additional dairy-free vegetable recipes can be found in Chapter 7.

Combine mayonnaise, vinegar, sugar, onion, salt, pepper, mustard, and tarragon. Toss with cabbage, green pepper, and carrots. Chill.

Makes 4 servings

Dairy-Free Cream Sauce

DAIRY-FREE
EGG-FREE

When you need to make a cream sauce for vegetables but cannot use milk because of a sensitivity, here's the sauce for you.

3 tablespoons dairy-free margarine
3 tablespoons flour
1 cup chicken broth

¼ teaspoon salt
⅛ teaspoon pepper
⅛ teaspoon tarragon

Melt margarine in a small saucepan. Add flour and stir over low heat until mixture is smooth and bubbly. Gradually stir in broth. Heat, stirring constantly, until mixture is thick. Add salt, pepper, and tarragon.

Makes 1 cup

Mayonnaise

GLUTEN-FREE
DAIRY-FREE

You'll never run out of mayonnaise again, once you have learned how to make your own in minutes. If it's too thin, drizzle extra oil into it until it is as thick as desired.

1 egg
½ teaspoon salt

2 tablespoons vinegar
1 cup salad oil

Break egg into electric blender container. Add salt and vinegar; blend. Add ⅓ cup salad oil; blend. Uncover and blend while pouring the remaining salad oil in a steady stream. Turn off when all oil is mixed in. Store in refrigerator in a tightly covered container.

Makes 1¼ cups

Potato Pancakes

DAIRY-FREE

Peanut oil gives these pancakes a special flavor. Cornstarch may be substituted for the flour, if necessary.

2 pounds potatoes, pared
1 onion
1 egg, lightly beaten
2 tablespoons flour
½ teaspoon salt
½ teaspoon pepper
1 cup peanut oil
Applesauce

Grate potatoes into a deep bowl. Grate onions and add to potatoes. Add beaten egg, flour, salt, and pepper and mix well. Heat oil in a large skillet. Drop large spoonfuls of mixture into the hot oil and fry as pancakes. Serve with applesauce.

Makes 6 servings

PASTA AND NOODLES

Pasta

DAIRY-FREE

Make your own pasta this easy way. Wider strips may be used to make lasagne.

1¼ cups flour
2 eggs
¼ teaspoon salt
1 tablespoon water

Place flour in a mound on a pastry board. Make a hole in the center; break eggs into the hole. Add salt and water. Mix with fingers until well blended into a dough, then knead until dough comes together easily and leaves your hands clean of bits. Let dough rest, covered, for 1 hour. Divide dough into 8 pieces. Roll paper-thin with pasta machine or with rolling pin. Cut by machine into desired widths or roll up and slice with a sharp knife. Spread out and dry for at least 20 minutes. Cook in boiling salted water for 10 minutes, or as directed in recipe.

Makes 4 servings

Spaghetti Milanese

DAIRY-FREE

This is an intriguing way to use chicken livers—chunked into an aromatic tomato sauce.

¼ cup salad oil
1 large onion, diced fine
1 cup sliced fresh mushrooms
2 cloves garlic, minced
8 chicken livers
1 teaspoon oregano
½ teaspoon salt
¼ teaspoon pepper
2 1-pound cans Italian tomatoes,
    packed in sauce with basil leaf
1 pound spaghetti

Heat oil in a skillet. Add diced onion, sliced mushrooms, and minced garlic; sauté until onions are golden. Cut livers into small chunks; add to skillet and brown on all sides. Add oregano, salt, and pepper. Add tomatoes, breaking with the edge of a spoon. Simmer for 15 minutes. Meanwhile, cook spaghetti as directed on package. Drain. Pour onto a warm platter. Pour sauce over and toss lightly to coat the pasta. Serve hot at once.

Makes 4–6 servings

Spaghetti with White Clam Sauce

DAIRY-FREE

No need to toss your pasta with butter. Here's the way to make it garlicky good.

2 6½-ounce cans minced
   clams
½ cup olive oil
3 cloves garlic, minced
½ teaspoon salt

2 tablespoons chopped
   parsley
¼ teaspoon pepper
1 pound spaghetti

Drain clams. Heat olive oil in a skillet. Add garlic and brown lightly. Add parsley, clams, salt, and pepper. Stir and simmer several minutes; remove from heat. Meanwhile, cook spaghetti according to package directions. Drain. Pour onto a warm platter and pour clam sauce over. Toss lightly and serve at once.

Makes 6 servings

Spaghetti with Tomato-Meat Sauce

DAIRY-FREE

If there is a beef sensitivity, use ground turkey in the sauce. Either way, it's a great way to stretch ½ pound of protein to feed a hungry sextet.

3 tablespoons olive oil
1 large onion, diced
1 green pepper, diced
½ pound chopped beef
2 1-pound cans Italian
   tomatoes

1 6-ounce can tomato paste
1 teaspoon salt
¼ teaspoon pepper
½ teaspoon oregano
1 pound spaghetti

Heat oil in a large skillet. Sauté onion and green pepper. Add ground beef and break into tiny bits with a fork; brown well. Stir in tomatoes and tomato paste. Add salt, pepper, and oregano. Simmer, covered, for 1 hour. Fifteen minutes before you are ready to serve, cook spaghetti according to directions on package. Drain. Place on a warm platter and pour tomato-meat sauce over pasta. Serve at once.

Makes 6 servings

Green Noodles with Spinach Sauce

DAIRY-FREE

Tofu can take on many dairy characteristics when used in a sauce. Here is a splendid way to serve it with spinach pasta.

1 1-pound package green noodles	2 cloves garlic, peeled
12 spinach leaves	½ teaspoon salt
4 sprigs parsley	½ cup broken walnuts
½ cup tofu	¼ cup olive oil
	½ cup hot water

Cook green noodles as directed on package; drain. Place all other ingredients in an electric blender and process into a fine sauce. Pour over cooked noodles and serve at once.

Makes 6 servings

Macaroni and Egg Salad

DAIRY-FREE

For those who think that macaroni only goes with cheese sauce, here's a peppier way to serve it.

1 tablespoon salt	¼ teaspoon dillweed
3 quarts boiling water	⅛ teaspoon pepper
2 cups elbow macaroni (8 ounces)	3 tablespoons vinegar
½ cup chopped celery	2 tablespoons salad oil
¼ cup chopped Bermuda onion	4 hard-cooked eggs
1 teaspoon salt	⅔ cup Mayonnaise (see recipe)
	Lettuce leaves

Add the 1 tablespoon salt to rapidly boiling water. Add macaroni gradually so that the water continues to boil. Cook uncovered, stirring occasionally, until tender. Drain. Rinse with cold water; drain again. Mix macaroni, celery, onion, 1 teaspoon salt, dillweed, pepper, vinegar, and oil in a large bowl. Chill. Peel and coarsely chop eggs and add with mayonnaise to the chilled macaroni mixture; mix lightly. Serve on lettuce.

Makes 4 servings

BREADS

Banana Walnut Muffins

DAIRY-FREE

So you thought dairy-free meant the end of bountiful muffins? Use soft bananas to make these mouthwatering delights.

2 eggs
⅓ cup corn oil
2 ripe bananas, mashed
1¾ cups unbleached flour
2 teaspoons baking powder
¾ teaspoon baking soda
½ teaspoon cinnamon
1 cup apple juice
1 cup chopped walnuts
½ cup raisins (optional)

Beat eggs until lemon-colored. Add oil and bananas and beat well. Combine flour, baking powder, baking soda, and cinnamon; add alternately to the batter with the apple juice. Stir in walnuts and raisins. Spoon into greased or paper-lined muffin tins. Bake at 350°F. 30 minutes or until browned.

Makes 12 large muffins

Dairy-Free White Bread

DAIRY-FREE

This dairy-free white bread will turn out delicious every time if you follow the directions with care. Dough is kneaded enough when you press it with a finger and the dough springs back, leaving only a slight indentation. Be sure to toast the leftover slices and process them into breadcrumbs for future use.

3 cups all purpose flour
1 package active dry yeast,
  ¼ ounce
1 tablespoon sugar
1 teaspoon salt
2 tablespoons softened
  dairy-free margarine
1⅛ cups hot tap water
Cooking oil

Combine 1 cup flour, undissolved yeast, sugar, and salt in a large bowl. Stir well to blend, then add margarine and hot tap water. Beat with an electric mixer for 2 minutes. Scrape sides. Add another cup of flour and beat on high speed for 1 minute until dough is thick and elastic. Add remaining flour, stirring it in with a wooden spoon; then remove dough onto a floured board. Knead for 10 minutes, until dough is smooth and elastic. Let rest 20 minutes on the board. Punch down and shape dough into a loaf to fit a 8½-by-4½-inch loaf pan. Place in the loaf pan and brush top lightly with cooking oil. Cover pan loosely with plastic wrap. Allow dough to rise, away from drafts, until double in bulk, about 1 hour. Preheat oven to 400° F., then bake bread for 30 to 40 minutes until lightly browned.

Makes 1 loaf (may be frozen for future use)

Pumpkin Bread

DAIRY-FREE

Pumpkin is not only for Thanksgiving—here's a way to serve it year-round. Try it with orange marmalade for an additional taste treat.

⅔ cup pure vegetable shortening	**1½ teaspoons salt**
2⅔ cups sugar	**1 teaspoon cinnamon**
4 eggs	**½ teaspoon baking powder**
1 1-pound can pumpkin	**1 orange**
⅔ cup water	**⅔ cup chopped nuts**
3⅓ cups flour	**⅔ cup chopped raisins or**
2 teaspoons baking soda	**dates**

Cream shortening and sugar thoroughly. Add eggs, beating well. Add pumpkin and water. Sift together flour, baking soda, salt, cinnamon, and baking powder; add to pumpkin mixture. Remove seeds from orange after cutting it into sections (do not remove rind). Using a food processor, blender, or grinder, grind orange and rind; add to pumpkin mixture. Stir in nuts and raisins. Pour into 2 well-greased 9-by-5-inch loaf pans and bake in a 350° F. oven for 1 hour.

Makes 2 loaves (may be frozen for future use)

Challah

DAIRY-FREE

This recipe makes two medium loaves of braided bread. It has a wholesome homemade texture with a shiny rich brown crust. Like Mama used to make!

6 cups unsifted, unbleached flour	**1 tablespoon sugar**
2 packages active dry yeast, ¼-ounce each	**2 teaspoons salt**
1⅓ cups warm water	**3 eggs**
	3 tablespoons corn oil
	Additional corn oil
	Poppy seeds

Sift the flour into a large bowl. Crumble the yeast into a small bowl; add warm water and sugar. When it bubbles after a few moments, add salt. Beat eggs and spoon off 1 tablespoon to use as a glaze for the loaves; add corn oil to the remaining beaten eggs and stir well. Then stir egg mixture into the yeast mixture and quickly stir the combined mixture into the flour until you have a soft ball. Knead this well, until smooth and elastic. Place in a large bowl, brush additional corn oil over top surface of dough, cover with plastic wrap and let rise in a warm place free from drafts, until double in bulk. Punch dough down and knead again. Divide the dough in half and divide each half into three parts. Form long fat ropes of the dough and braid three ropes loosely together. Repeat with second group of three ropes. Place each braid into a 9-by-5-inch loaf pan. Let rise again for ½ hour. Brush with reserved beaten egg and sprinkle with poppy seeds. Bake in a preheated 400° F. oven for 45 minutes, or until richly browned.

Makes 2 loaves

DESSERTS

Apple Crisp

DAIRY-FREE
EGG-FREE

Use uncooked cream of rice cereal in place of the flour to make this recipe gluten-free; add an extra tablespoon of shortening to keep it soft.

6 tart apples, peeled
   and sliced thin
2 tablespoons lemon juice
1 cup sugar

¾ teaspoon cinnamon
¼ teaspoon nutmeg
1 cup flour
⅓ cup shortening

Toss sliced apples with lemon juice in a bowl. Combine sugar, cinnamon, and nutmeg; add ½ cup of this mixture to the apples. Mix well. Spread the apples in a 9-inch square baking pan. Add flour and shortening to the remaining sugar mixture; work through until crumbly. Sprinkle this mixture over the apples. Bake in a 350°F. oven for 45–50 minutes, or until apples are tender and topping is browned and crisp.

Makes 6 servings

Angel Food Cake

DAIRY-FREE

What to do with the egg yolks left over from this recipe? Make Hollandaise Sauce (see recipe) or substitute 2 egg yolks for each egg in Mayonnaise (see recipe).

12 egg whites
¼ teaspoon salt
1 teaspoon cream of tartar
1¼ cups sugar

1 cup confectioners' sugar
1¼ cups cake flour
1 tablespoon lemon juice

Preheat oven to 350°F. Let egg whites come to room temperature to get the greatest volume; add salt and beat until foamy. Add cream of tartar and beat until soft peaks form. Sift together sugar, confectioners' sugar, and cake flour; fold into egg whites. Fold in lemon juice. Pour into an ungreased 10-inch tube pan and bake for 50–60 minutes. Remove from oven and invert tube onto the neck of an empty soda bottle, hanging the cake upside down to cool. This will prevent it from collapsing.

Makes one 10-inch cake, about 10 servings

Banana Chiffon Cake

DAIRY-FREE

Here's another way to use up those too-soft bananas. Turn them into cake and watch them disappear!

2½ cups sifted wheat flour	½ cup salad oil
¾ cup sugar	5 eggs, separated
¾ cup light brown sugar	⅓ cup cold water
1 tablespoon baking powder	1⅓ cups mashed bananas
1 teaspoon salt	1 teaspoon pure vanilla
½ teaspoon allspice	extract

Sift flour, sugar, brown sugar, baking powder, salt, and allspice into a mixing bowl. Add oil, egg yolks, water, bananas, and vanilla and beat until smooth. In a separate bowl, beat egg whites until stiff peaks form. Fold into batter just until blended. Pour into an ungreased 10-inch tube pan and bake in a 325°F. oven for 55 minutes. Then increase temperature to 350°F. and bake 15–20 minutes longer, or until a cake tester inserted in the center comes out clean. Invert tube onto the neck of an empty soda bottle and let cool.

Makes 16 slices

Carrot Pudding

DAIRY-FREE
GLUTEN-FREE

What a wonderful way to get vitamin C into the diet. A food processor makes the shredding a cinch, if you don't feel like taking the time to do it with a hand grater.

3 eggs, separated	1 teaspoon grated orange rind
3 tablespoons sugar	¼ teaspoon dried dillweed
¼ cup orange juice	3 cups shredded raw carrots
¼ teaspoon salt	

Beat egg yolks with sugar until light and fluffy. Gradually add orange juice. Stir in salt, orange rind, dillweed and carrots. Beat egg whites until stiff but not dry; fold into carrot batter. Turn into a buttered 1½-quart casserole. Bake in a 350°F. oven for 30 minutes.

Makes 6 servings

Cocoa Chiffon Cake

DAIRY-FREE

Be sure to use the fine cake flour that has baking powder added if you want a delicately porous chiffon cake. Don't use a cocoa mix—pure cocoa is needed here.

1½ cups sifted cake flour
1½ cups sugar
¼ cup cocoa
1 teaspoon baking soda
1 teaspoon salt
7 eggs, separated
½ cup salad oil
¾ cup water
1 teaspoon pure vanilla extract
½ teaspoon cream of tartar

Sift flour, ½ cup of the sugar, cocoa, baking soda, and salt into a small mixing bowl. Add egg yolks, oil, water, and vanilla. Beat at low speed until blended. Beat at medium speed until smooth, about 2 minutes. Beat egg whites until foamy; add cream of tartar and beat until soft peaks form. Gradually add the remaining 1 cup of sugar, beating well after each addition. Fold in the egg yolk mixture. Pour batter into an ungreased 10-inch tube pan. Bake in a preheated 325° F. oven for 55 minutes. Increase temperature to 350° F. and bake an additional 10 minutes. Invert tube onto the neck of an empty soda bottle and let cool.

Makes 12–16 servings

Dairy-Free Pastry

DAIRY-FREE
EGG-FREE

When you need a flaky nondairy pastry for pie or individual tarts, here's the best way to put it together.

2 cups flour	**⅔ cup pure vegetable shortening**
1 teaspoon salt	**4–5 tablespoons cold water**

Mix flour, salt, and shortening together, using a pastry blender or two forks, until it looks like coarse cornmeal. Slowly pour water over and work in. Refrigerate at least one hour. Then roll half the dough into a crust, using a floured board and floured rolling pin. Roll the other half into a second crust. Place one crust in a pie pan, fill with the desired filling, and top with the remaining crust. Crimp edges together to seal. If making a one-crust pie shell, place the second crust in another pan and freeze until needed; or halve the recipe and prepare only one crust.

Makes 2 9-inch crusts

Apple-Nut Bars

DAIRY-FREE

If you plan to stop for a few minutes after chopping the apples, be sure to sprinkle them with lemon juice to prevent natural browning.

2 peeled apples, cored and cut into pieces	**1 egg**
¾ cup sifted flour	**¼ cup orange juice**
1 teaspoon baking powder	**¾ cup light brown sugar**
½ teaspoon cinnamon	**1 teaspoon pure vanilla extract**
¼ teaspoon salt	**½ cup peanut butter**

Place apples in a blender or food processor and chop fine (or chop in a wooden bowl by hand). Combine flour, baking powder, cinnamon, and salt in a bowl; add chopped apples. Place egg, orange juice, brown sugar, and vanilla in the blender and process until well mixed; add peanut butter and process again. Pour into apple mixture and stir well. Pour into a greased 8-inch square pan. Bake at 350°F. for 25–30 minutes. Cut into 2-inch bars.

Makes 16 bars

Coconut-Peanut Bars

DAIRY-FREE

To make a crunchier topping, sprinkle additional coconut over the top of the batter—it's a delicious dairy-free mouthful.

1 cup sifted flour
1 teaspoon baking powder
¼ teaspoon salt
⅓ cup salad oil
½ cup creamy or chunk-style peanut butter
1 cup sugar
2 eggs, beaten
1 teaspoon pure vanilla extract
1 cup shredded coconut, chopped

Grease a 9-by-9-by-2-inch baking pan. Sift together flour, baking powder, and salt. Mix oil and peanut butter in a bowl. Stir in sugar, eggs, and vanilla. Add flour mixture, beating until smooth. Fold in coconut. Turn into prepared pan, spreading to cover bottom evenly. Bake in a 350°F. oven about 30 minutes, or until slightly browned. Cut into 3-by-1-inch bars while warm.

Makes 2 dozen bars

Lemon Crullers

DAIRY-FREE

These crullers are best served hot and fresh. Be sure the oil is bubbling hot so the batter solidifies and puffs up quickly.

1 egg

1 tablespoon grated lemon
   rind

¼ cup sugar

1 tablespoon water

2 tablespoons corn oil

2 teaspoons lemon juice

1¼ cups flour

1 teaspoon baking powder

⅛ teaspoon salt

Granulated or confectioners'
   sugar (optional)

Beat egg until lemon-colored. Add lemon rind, sugar, water, oil, and lemon juice; beat well. Add flour, baking powder, and salt; mix well. Drop rounded tablespoonfuls of dough into bubbling cooking oil. The crullers will puff and brown at once; turn and brown the other side. Remove from oil and drain on paper towels. Roll in granulated or confectioners' sugar, if desired.

Makes 18 crullers

Ladyfingers

DAIRY-FREE

Ladyfingers are dainty to nibble at teatime or to use as a framework for a charlotte dessert. Special ladyfinger pans are available at gourmet shops and restaurant supply stores.

6 eggs

1¼ cups sugar

1 teaspoon pure vanilla
   extract

1 cup sifted cake flour

⅓ cup cornstarch

¼ teaspoon salt

Grease and lightly flour ladyfinger pans. Beat together eggs, 1 cup of the sugar, and vanilla on medium-high speed of electric mixer until light, lemon-colored, and double in bulk. Sift together flour, cornstarch, and salt. Gradually fold into beaten egg mixture, mixing well. Fill each ladyfinger pan with about 2 tablespoons of batter. When all are filled, sprinkle with about 1 tablespoon of sugar per dozen ladyfingers. Keep remaining batter refrigerated while baking first batch. Bake in 350° F. oven for 12–15 minutes, or until a cake tester inserted in the center comes out clean. Cool slightly, remove from pan; cool on rack.

Makes about 4 dozen

NOTE: Recipe may be cut in half. Use 3 tablespoons cornstarch.

Wafers

DAIRY-FREE

Except for the egg yolks, there is no fat in this recipe. The recipe makes dozens of flat cookies that are wafer-thin.

½ cup flour
2 tablespoons cornstarch
⅛ teaspoon salt
2 egg whites
2 egg yolks, lightly beaten
½ cup sugar
¾ teaspoon pure vanilla extract

Sift flour, cornstarch, and salt together; set aside. Beat egg whites until soft peaks form when beaters are raised. Beat in egg yolks, then sugar. Blend in sifted dry ingredients. Stir in vanilla extract. Drop by teaspoonfuls onto greased baking sheet 2 inches apart. Bake in 400°F. oven for 8–10 minutes, or until golden brown in center with a slightly darker brown edge.

Makes 4 dozen

Coconut-Peanut Macaroons

DAIRY-FREE

Each macaroon is a mouthful of fluff with a peanut flavor and a crunch of coconut. A dairy-free delight!

3 egg whites	½ cup creamy peanut butter
1 cup sugar	1 cup shredded coconut
1 tablespoon flour	

Beat egg whites until foamy. Gradually add sugar and continue to beat until egg whites are stiff and thick. Fold in flour. Fold meringue into peanut butter. Fold in coconut. Drop by tablespoonfuls onto ungreased cookie sheet covered with brown paper. Bake in a 325°F. oven for 20–25 minutes. Remove from paper when cool.

Makes approximately 3 dozen

Peanut Butter Kisses

DAIRY-FREE
GLUTEN-FREE

This version of a merinque cookie is made without any flour. Be sure that the whites are beaten so stiff that the peaks stand up in the bowl.

2 egg whites	⅔ cup sugar
⅛ teaspoon cream of tartar	½ cup chunky peanut butter

Beat egg whites and cream of tartar together until stiff peaks form. Add sugar, 1 tablespoon at a time, beating well after each addition. Continue beating until very stiff peaks form. Lightly fold in peanut butter just until mixed through. Drop by teaspoonfuls onto a greased cookie sheet. Bake in a slow (300°F.) oven for 25 minutes, or until lightly browned. Immediately remove from cookie sheet.

Makes about 3 dozen

Peanut Butter Wheat Crackers

DAIRY-FREE
EGG-FREE

Make your own crackers without any milk or eggs. The peanut butter gives an interesting flavor, and the caraway seeds make them crunchy.

1 cup unsifted unbleached flour
1 cup unsifted whole wheat flour
¼ cup wheat germ
1½ teaspoons caraway seeds
1 teaspoon salt
½ teaspoon baking soda
1 cup chunky peanut butter
about ½ cup water
2 tablespoons cider vinegar

In a large bowl mix together flour, whole wheat flour, wheat germ, caraway seeds, salt, and baking soda. With a pastry blender or two knives, cut in peanut butter until coarse crumbs form. Add water and vinegar; mix until dough holds together. If mixture is too dry, add additional water 1 tablespoon at a time. Divide dough in half. On lightly floured surface, roll half of dough out to ⅛-inch thickness. Cut with 3-inch round cookie cutter. Repeat with scraps and remaining half of dough. Place on an ungreased cookie sheet. Brush surface with water. Bake for 13–15 minutes in a 375°F. oven, until browned and crisp. Remove from pan and cool on wire racks. Store in airtight container.

Makes about 40

Peanut Butter Cookies

DAIRY-FREE

Dough can be rolled into wax paper and sliced ¼-inch thick, if desired. Dough may also be frozen for future use.

1 cup peanut butter	**1 egg**
½ cup shortening	**½ teaspoon vanilla**
½ cup sugar	**1½ cups sifted flour**
½ cup brown sugar	**1 teaspoon baking powder**

Beat peanut butter and shortening together until creamy; add sugars slowly and continue to beat until fluffy. Add egg and vanilla; beat well. Add flour and baking powder; mix well. Form into 1-inch balls and place on a greased cookie sheet. Flatten each ball with the tines of a fork, leaving a crosshatch pattern on the dough. Bake for 10 minutes in a 350°F. oven.

Makes 4 dozen

Quick Peanut Butter Cookies

DAIRY-FREE
GLUTEN-FREE

Here's a four-ingredient mouthful of goodness for the dairy-sensitive. Store in a tightly covered tin to keep fresh longer.

1 cup chunky peanut butter	**1 egg**
1 cup sugar	**1 teaspoon vanilla**

Beat peanut butter and sugar together. Add egg and vanilla and blend well. Shape dough into 1-inch balls and place about 2 inches apart on an ungreased cookie sheet. Flatten slightly with a fork. Bake in a 325°F. oven for 15–20 minutes, or until golden brown and cookies spring back when touched lightly.

Makes about 3 dozen

Zucchini Oatmeal Cookies

DAIRY-FREE

There's something virtuous about grating a vegetable into a cookie. Here it is combined with some breakfast cereal as well.

1 egg
½ cup corn oil
½ cup sugar
½ cup brown sugar
1 cup flour
½ teaspoon baking soda
¼ teaspoon salt
¼ teaspoon cinnamon
¼ teaspoon nutmeg
1¼ cups rolled oats
1 cup grated fresh zucchini

Beat egg, corn oil, sugar, and brown sugar together until well blended. Combine flour, baking soda, salt, cinnamon, and nutmeg; add to egg mixture. Add oats and zucchini and mix well. Drop ¼-cup portions onto a greased baking sheet one inch apart; flatten with the back of a spoon. Bake in a preheated 350°F. oven for 12 minutes, or until edges are lightly browned.

Makes 12 large cookies (or 4 dozen if dropped by tablespoonfuls)

5
The
Egg-Free
Diet

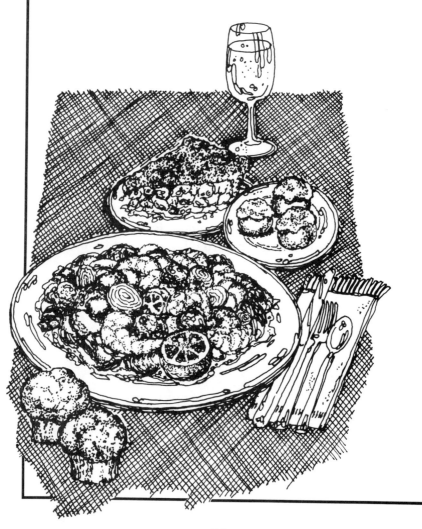

When you suspect or have been advised that you have an allergy to eggs you must completely eliminate eggs from the diet. Eggs are easy enough to avoid in their whole form, such as scrambled eggs, poached eggs, and boiled eggs. You must realize, however, that eggs are hidden in many other foods that don't feature them. Therefore, it is necessary to become acquainted with those foods that are likely to contain eggs so that you can avoid them as well.

An obvious use for eggs is in baked goods. Since eggs are used as a leavening agent in baking, you can assume that every kind of bread, muffin, cake, and cookie has egg in it. You will find recipes in this chapter that are eggless, using other ingredients to substitute for leavening. Otherwise, you will have to omit all commercially baked products, unless you are sure that they are egg-free.

Commercial products to avoid include pancake mixes, cake mixes, batter bread mixes, and all cookie and muffin mixes. In restaurants, do not order any fried foods that have been dipped into batter or breaded, because most batters contain eggs and most breaded foods have been dipped into an egg mixture before being breaded. Even if your fried order does not have any egg in it, the cooking oil may have been contaminated with egg. Thus, if you order French fried potatoes that are cooked in the same oil as the breaded items in a restaurant, your order may come in contact with residuals of egg from another order. Therefore, check whether the potatoes are fried in a separate unit—as is the case in larger cooking establishments.

Eggs are also used as an emulsifier in many food products, such as mayonnaise, salad dressings, sauces, and malted cocoa drinks. Suspect any mayonnaise-type dressing—hollandaise sauce, thousand island dressing, tartar sauce, and Russian dressing—of containing egg. Use only oil-and-vinegar-based dressings, unless you are sure that there is no egg in the product.

Eggs are also used in the making of ice cream, ices, pasta, and marshmallows. Some cooks use eggshells to clear coffee, so ask before you drink.

Read labels very carefully to be sure that dried egg is not listed as an ingredient of anything that will be served to the egg-sensitive person.

Since you are eliminating a very important source of protein in the diet, be sure that it is replaced with other protein foods. Eggs also are an important source of vitamins and minerals that are essential to human development and continued well-being. The egg yolk, for instance, is a rich source of choline and biotin (one of the B-complex vitamins). Eggs provide vitamins A, B_2, D, niacin, and E. Also, copper, iron, phosphorous, and both saturated and unsaturated fats are contained in eggs.

This chapter has been designed to help you create recipes that are totally free of eggs. For additional egg-free recipes, refer both to the index and to Chapter 7 for multiple-allergy recipes.

APPETIZERS

Creamy Dip

EGG-FREE
GLUTEN-FREE

If a zestier taste is desired, add some white horseradish or a few drops of Worcestershire sauce. Some cooks may want to add both!

1 cup dairy sour cream
1 teaspoon grated onion
1 teaspoon salt
½ teaspoon grated lemon rind
1½ tablespoons lemon juice
¼ teaspoon pure soy sauce

Beat sour cream until light and fluffy. Add the remaining ingredients and mix well. Chill.

Makes 1⅛ cup

Date-Nut Spread

EGG-FREE
GLUTEN-FREE

This spread will go well with rice crackers for a gluten-free muncher. Otherwise, fill celery stalks with the mixture and serve as an hors d'oeuvre.

1 cup cottage cheese
½ cup finely chopped dates
½ cup raisins

⅓ cup chopped pecans
½ teaspoon salt

Beat cottage cheese in a small bowl until fairly smooth. Stir in dates, raisins, nuts, and salt.

Makes about 1⅔ cups

Liptauer Cheese

EGG-FREE
GLUTEN-FREE

Here's a wonderful party spread with intriguing ingredients. Serve on sliced cucumber rounds for those who have multiple allergies.

Butter to coat 2-cup bowl
2 tablespoons dried parsley flakes
1 cup butter, softened
1 8-ounce package cream cheese, softened
3 anchovy fillets, chopped
1 teaspoon dry mustard
1 teaspoon paprika
1 teaspoon finely chopped onion
1 teaspoon chopped capers
1 teaspoon chopped chives
1 teaspoon finely chopped parsley
½ teaspoon caraway seeds

Coat the inside of a 2-cup bowl with butter; sprinkle with parsley flakes to cover all sides. In a separate bowl, stir softened butter into softened cream cheese until well mixed. Add anchovies, mustard, paprika, onion, capers, chives, parsley, and caraway seeds. Press the mixture into the coated bowl. Chill 4 hours or until firm. Unmold before serving.

Makes 2 cups

Tuna-Cheese Spread

EGG-FREE

Tuna fish has a way of pleasing most everyone. This spread shows you how to get a lot of gourmet mileage from one can.

1 7-ounce can water-packed tuna, drained and flaked
¼ cup cottage cheese
¼ cup plain yogurt
2 tablespoons finely chopped onion
1 teaspoon white horseradish
¼ teaspoon pure Worcestershire sauce
Melba toast rounds or egg-free crackers

Mix the tuna and cottage cheese together. Add yogurt, onion, horseradish, and Worcestershire sauce. Mix well. Chill. Spread on crackers or place in a bowl for do-it-yourself spreading.

Makes 1½ cups (enough for 36 crackers)

Guacamole

EGG-FREE
GLUTEN-FREE

A ripe avocado should feel soft to the touch. Otherwise, let it ripen at room temperature before using it in this dip.

2 ripe avocados, mashed fine
¼ cup dairy sour cream
2 tablespoons grated onion
1 tomato, pèeled and chopped fine
1 clove garlic, minced fine
1 tablespoon lemon juice
1 teaspoon salt
½ teaspoon chili powder

Combine all ingredients and mix well. Cover and chill for several hours.

Makes about 2½ cups

Cheese-Stuffed Mushrooms

EGG-FREE/
GLUTEN-FREE

Cold stuffed mushrooms are easy to prepare ahead of time and provide a marvelous mouthful.

24 large fresh mushrooms
½ cup cottage cheese
½ teaspoon garlic sauce
1 tablespoon chopped chives

¼ teaspoon Worcestershire
  sauce
¼ teaspoon thyme
Paprika

Wash mushrooms; remove stems and reserve for another use. Cover mushroom caps with salted water and boil in a covered saucepan for 15 minutes. Drain and chill. Combine cottage cheese, garlic salt, chives, Worcestershire sauce, and thyme; mix well. Spoon into mushroom caps. Sprinkle with paprika. Serve chilled.

Makes 2 dozen

Apricot Cheese Ball

EGG-FREE

This cheese ball can be made gluten-free by eliminating the bran buds and rolling in chopped nuts instead.

1 8-ounce package cream cheese,
  softened
½ cup pot cheese or dry-curd
  cottage cheese
2 tablespoons chopped dried
  apricots

1 tablespoon grated onion
1 teaspoon lemon juice
½ teaspoon salt
½ teaspoon curry powder
½ cup bran buds cereal

Beat cream cheese and pot cheese together until smooth. Stir in apricots, onion, lemon juice, salt, and curry powder. Chill until stiff enough to shape into a ball. Roll ball in bran buds cereal. Chill. Serve with crackers.

Makes 1 cheese ball 4" diameter

Pimiento Cheese Ball

EGG-FREE
GLUTEN-FREE

Chopped pimientos give this otherwise white cheese ball a shot of color throughout. Serve in a bed of parsley sprigs for a wreath-like effect.

½ pound white cheddar
   cheese, grated
2 3-ounce packages
   cream cheese
1 clove garlic, crushed

2 drained pimientos,
   chopped fine
2 tablespoons grated onion
Paprika

Combine cheddar and cream cheese. Add pimientos, garlic, and onion; mix well. Form into a ball. Sprinkle a thick coating of paprika over entire surface. Chill until ready to serve. Serve as a spread for celery or crackers that don't contain allergens.
Makes 1 pound (enough for 24 servings)

Salmon Cheese Log

EGG-FREE
GLUTEN-FREE

There is nothing wooden about the taste of this salmon log. And it's incredibly spreadable!

1 16-ounce can red salmon
1 8-ounce package cream
   cheese
2 tablespoons lemon juice
1 teaspoon grated lemon
   rind

1 teaspoon grated onion
1 teaspoon white horseradish
½ cup chopped pecans
¼ cup chopped fresh parsley
Celery sticks

Drain salmon and remove bones and skin; mash. Blend with cream cheese, lemon juice, lemon rind, onion, and horseradish. Chill until firm. Form into a log. Combine pecans and parsley; roll log in this mixture to coat well. Chill again until ready to serve. Serve with celery sticks or crackers.

Makes about 24 servings

Shrimp Balls

EGG-FREE
GLUTEN-FREE

An easy way to cook shrimp is to bring water to a boil and drop the shrimp in. When the water boils again, cover tightly, turn the heat off, and leave the shrimp in for at least 30 minutes. As the pot cools, the shrimp will be cooked to perfection.

½ pound shrimp, cooked, shelled, and cleaned
1 3-ounce package cream cheese
¼ cup finely diced celery
2 teaspoons grated onion
1 teaspoon white horseradish
¼ teaspoon Worcestershire sauce
¼ teaspoon salt
¼ cup finely chopped fresh parsley

Chop shrimp very fine. Mash cream cheese until soft and fluffy; add chopped shrimp. Add celery, onion, horseradish, Worcestershire sauce, and salt. Form into ½-inch balls. Roll in chopped parsley. Chill.

Makes about 2 dozen hors d'oeuvres

Pizza Wedges

EGG-FREE

Add some sliced mushrooms or green peppers to dress up these pizza snacks.

1 cup pure tomato sauce
1 tablespoon olive oil
½ teaspoon oregano
4 English muffins, split
1 8-ounce package mozzarella cheese slices
3 tablespoons grated Parmesan cheese

Combine tomato sauce, olive oil, and oregano. Arrange English muffin halves on an ungreased cookie sheet. Spoon tomato sauce mixture onto each muffin half; top with a slice of mozzarella cheese and sprinkle with Parmesan cheese. Broil for about 3 minutes, or until cheese is melted and lightly browned. Cut each muffin half into quarters.

Makes 32 wedges—4–6 servings

SOUPS

Cream of Spinach Soup

EGG-FREE

The thick, white sauce may be made with 1 tablespoon of cornstarch, in place of the 2 tablespoons of wheat flour, for the gluten-sensitive.

1 10-ounce package frozen chopped spinach	¼ teaspoon nutmeg
1 small onion, diced fine	2 tablespoons butter
1 cup water	2 tablespoons wheat flour
½ teaspoon salt	3 cups milk

Place spinach, onion, water, salt, and nutmeg in a saucepan. Cover and cook for 20 minutes, until very tender. Push mixture through a sieve or puree in an electric blender. Melt butter in a small saucepan; stir in flour and cook until thick and bubbling. Remove from heat and stir in milk; return to heat and cook until thickened. Add spinach mixture. Serve hot.

Makes 4–6 servings

Cream of Mushroom Soup

EGG-FREE

Use half as much cornstarch as wheat flour when making a substitution for thickening soups and sauces. Float some chopped chives on the top for garnish.

2 tablespoons butter	2 cups Chicken Broth
1 tablespoon grated onion	(see recipe)
¼ teaspoon celery seed	2 tablespoons wheat flour
¼ pound fresh mushrooms, sliced	2 cups milk
2 tablespoons butter	½ teaspoon salt
	⅛ teaspoon pepper

Melt 2 tablespoons of butter in a saucepan; add grated onion, celery seed, and sliced mushrooms. Cook and stir until mush-rooms are limp. Add chicken broth and simmer 10 minutes. In a small saucepan, melt 2 tablespoons of butter and stir in flour until thick and bubbling. Remove from heat and stir in milk; return to heat and cook, stirring constantly, until thickened. Gradually stir thickened mixture into mushroom mixture until smooth. Heat and serve.

Makes 4 servings

Cream of Celery Soup

EGG-FREE

A food processor can make fast work of celery chopping. For extra celery flavor, add a dash of celery seed.

1 bunch celery
1 quart water
1 onion, diced fine
1 teaspoon salt
¼ teaspoon nutmeg
¼ teaspoon celery salt
¼ teaspoon cayenne pepper
3 tablespoons butter
3 tablespoons flour
2 cups milk

Chop celery fine, after trimming well. Place in a deep sauce-pan; add water, onion, salt, nutmeg, celery salt, and cayenne pepper. Bring to a boil, then reduce heat and simmer until celery and onion are soft and tender. Melt butter; stir in flour and then milk. Cook for several minutes, stirring constantly. Stir this mixture into the celery mixture and simmer for 5 minutes, stirring until smooth.

Makes 8–10 servings

Cream of Tomato Soup

EGG-FREE

This soup can be creamed with dairy-free margarine and 1½ tablespoons of cornstarch, if desired, making it suitable for those with multiple allergies. Float some popped corn on the top for an interesting garnish.

1 1-pound can tomatoes in natural juice	¼ teaspoon cayenne pepper
1 small onion, sliced	1 teaspoon Worcestershire sauce
1 sprig parsley	4 cups water
1 bay leaf	3 tablespoons butter
1 teaspoon salt	3 tablespoons flour

Empty tomatoes into a saucepan. Add sliced onion, parsley, bay leaf, salt, cayenne pepper, Worcestershire sauce, and water. Cook for 20 minutes. Press through a sieve or food mill. Melt butter in a small saucepan; add flour and stir until smooth. Pour some of the tomato soup into the butter-flour mixture and stir until very smooth; then gradually return this mixture to the tomato soup, stirring constantly. Heat and stir for several minutes before serving.

Makes 6 servings

Cod Chowder

EGG-FREE
GLUTEN-FREE

Start the meal with this stick-to-the-ribs chowder, then follow with a vegetable platter for a well-balanced meal.

1½ pounds fillet of cod	2 tablespoons butter
1 large onion, diced	½ teaspoon salt
2 large potatoes, diced	¼ teaspoon pepper
2 stalks celery, diced fine	¼ teaspoon thyme
1 quart milk	2 tablespoons cornstarch

Place fish in a large saucepan; cover with water and cook until fish falls apart easily. Add onion, potatoes, and celery; simmer until tender. Add milk, butter, salt, pepper, and thyme. Simmer and stir until butter is melted. Mix cornstarch with just enough water to make a smooth thin paste; spoon some of the hot soup liquid into this paste and then return the entire mixture to the soup, stirring constantly. Continue to stir and cook until soup thickens slightly. Then serve at once.

Makes 8–10 servings

Oyster Chowder

EGG-FREE
GLUTEN-FREE

When oysters are in season, this easy-to-make chowder will bring pearls of praise to the cook!

½ pint shucked oysters with liquid
2 cups milk
2 tablespoons sweet butter
1 small onion, diced fine
1 stalk celery, diced fine
2 potatoes, peeled and diced
2 cups water
½ teaspoon salt
¼ teaspoon pepper
¼ teaspoon celery seeds

Combine oysters, liquid, and milk; set aside. Melt butter in a saucepan; sauté onion and celery until limp. Add potatoes, water, salt, pepper, and celery seeds. Cover and simmer until vegetables are tender. Add oyster mixture: simmer 5 minutes.

Makes 4 servings

Onion Soup

EGG-FREE
GLUTEN-FREE

Omit the cheese and use dairy-free margarine with the onions, and you'll have a perfect offering for the milk-sensitive diner.

4 large sweet onions,
  sliced thin
3 tablespoons sweet butter
1 tablespoon salad oil
½ teaspoon salt

¼ teaspoon cayenne
1 quart Chicken Broth
  (see recipe)
Grated Parmesan cheese

Sauté onions in butter and oil until translucent. Add salt and cayenne pepper. Add chicken broth; cover and simmer for 20 minutes. Serve with grated Parmesan cheese.

Makes 4 servings

Potato Soup

EGG-FREE
GLUTEN-FREE

For a lovely way to serve potatoes, use a colorful soup bowl or sprinkle with extra fresh dillweed.

3 large potatoes, diced
1 leek or small onion,
  diced fine
2 stalks celery, diced fine
½ teaspoon salt

⅛ teaspoon pepper
½ teaspoon dried dillweed
1 quart milk
2 tablespoons butter
2 tablespoons cornstarch

Put diced potato, leek or onion, celery, salt, pepper, and dillweed into a large saucepan; barely cover with water and cook until potatoes are soft. Add milk and butter; simmer and stir until butter is melted. Stir cornstarch with just enough water to make a smooth, thin paste; spoon some of the hot soup liquid into this paste and then return the entire mixture to the soup, stirring constantly. Continue to stir and cook until soup thickens; do not let it boil.

Makes 8 servings

ENTREES

Beef

Muffin-Burgers

EGG-FREE

Omit the cheese and make sure you use egg-free/dairy-free breadcrumbs, and this recipe also becomes dairy-free.

1½ pounds ground beef
1½ cups egg-free breadcrumbs (see note below)
1 teaspoon minced onion
1 teaspoon salt
½ teaspoon dry mustard
1 cup applesauce (with no artificial additives)
3 slices white American cheese, quartered

Combine ground beef, breadcrumbs, onion, salt, and mustard in a large bowl. Toss together and add the applesauce. Mix thoroughly with a wooden spoon and let stand until the applesauce has moistened the ingredients thoroughly. Divide the meat mixture into 12 equal portions and pack into ungreased muffin cups. Bake in a preheated 350° F. oven for 15–20 minutes. Top each muffin-burger with a cheese wedge (omit for dairy-free); return to oven until cheese is slightly melted.

Makes 12 burgers

NOTE: For the bread in this recipe, use white bread or egg-free Whole Wheat Bread (see recipes), or choose another egg-free bread recipe from this book (see index).

Eggplant Parmigiana

EGG-FREE
GLUTEN-FREE

The dairy-sensitive can prepare this recipe without the grated cheese. Sprinkle with extra oregano instead.

1 pound lean ground beef
½ teaspoon salt
½ teaspoon dried ground oregano
¼ teaspoon pepper
¼ cup grated onion
1 6-ounce can tomato paste
1½ cups water
1 eggplant
¼ cup grated Parmesan cheese

Brown beef in a large skillet by breaking into crumbling pieces as it cooks. Add salt, oregano, pepper, and grated onion. Add tomato paste. Stir in water. Cover and simmer for 10 minutes. Meanwhile, peel eggplant and slice lengthwise into ¼-inch slices. Spoon a thin layer of the meat sauce into a flat baking dish. Arrange a single layer of eggplant slices over sauce. Top with another layer of sauce, then another layer of eggplant slices, and finally a last layer of sauce. Sprinkle with Parmesan cheese. Bake in a 350°F. oven for 35 minutes, or until eggplant is fork-tender.

Makes 6 servings

Flank Steak with Chive Butter

EGG-FREE
GLUTEN-FREE

Use dairy-free margarine for those allergic to milk. Any kind of mustard will do, but Dijon mustard has an extra flair.

1 flank steak, about 2 pounds   2 tablespoons butter, melted
1 teaspoon pure Dijon mustard   1 teaspoon chopped chives

Place flank steak on a broiling pan; spread a thin coating of mustard over top of steak. Broil for 5–6 minutes; turn and broil on the other side for an additional 5–6 minutes, or until done as desired. Combine melted butter and chives; pour over steak just before serving. To serve, slice very thinly on the diagonal, across the grain of the meat.

Makes 4 servings

Veal

Veal Marsala

EGG-FREE

To make this gluten-free, use cornstarch instead of flour for dredging. Dairy-free margarine may also be substituted for the butter, if desired.

1 pound thinly sliced veal
¼ cup flour
2 tablespoons olive oil
1 tablespoon butter
½ cup Marsala wine
1 tablespoon chopped parsley
¼ pound sliced fresh mushrooms

Lightly dredge veal slices in flour. Heat olive oil and butter in a heavy skillet. Sauté veal slices until lightly brown. Turn and lightly brown other side. Turn heat very low. Pour the wine over the veal and sprinkle with chopped parsley. Cover and simmer for 10 minutes or until tender. Serve at once.

Makes 4 servings

Veal Parmigiana

EGG-FREE

When you can't use an egg-dip before breading veal chops, prepare it this way with milk.

4 pieces thinly sliced veal cutlets, about 1½ pounds
¼ cup milk
½ cup egg-free breadcrumbs
1 tablespoon chopped parsley
¼ teaspoon paprika
3 tablespoons cooking oil
1 8-ounce can tomato sauce
4 thin slices mozzarella cheese

Dip each slice of veal in flat bowl containing the milk. Then dip in a mixture of breadcrumbs, parsley, and paprika; coat well. Heat oil in a skillet. Brown veal on both sides. Drain excess oil from the skillet. Pour tomato sauce over veal. Top with slices of cheese. Cover skillet and cook over low heat for several minutes, until the cheese melts.

Makes 4 servings

Veal Piccata

EGG-FREE
DAIRY-FREE

Those who are sensitive to gluten may substitute cornstarch for flour. This dish should be cooked just before serving to prevent sogginess.

2 pounds veal scallops
¼ cup flour
½ teaspoon salt
¼ teaspoon pepper
3 tablespoons oil
2 lemons
2 tablespoons chopped fresh parsley

Pound veal slices very thin. Dredge in combined flour, salt, and pepper. Heat oil in a large skillet. Sauté veal in oil, browning both sides. Add the juice of 1 lemon and slice the other lemon paper-thin; add slices to the skillet. Add parsley. Cover and simmer over low heat for 5 minutes more.

Makes 6 servings

Veal Paprikash

EGG-FREE

Nondairy margarine or oil may be substituted for the butter. Cornstarch will do just as well as flour.

2 pounds veal, cut into cubes
3 tablespoons butter
1 onion, diced fine
1 tablespoon sweet paprika
¼ cup flour
1 cup chicken broth
Hot rice or noodles (optional)

Trim veal of excess fat and set aside. Melt butter in a large skillet; add onion and sauté for several minutes. Add paprika. Lightly coat veal with flour and add to the skillet, turning to brown all sides. Add chicken broth and cover skillet; cook over low heat for 20 minutes, or until tender. Serve on hot rice or noodles, if desired.

Makes 8 servings

Pork

Stuffed Pork Chops

EGG-FREE

If allergic to pork, use veal or lamb chops instead and roast for just 45 minutes, or until tender. Use oil instead of butter, and dried bread made from a milk-free recipe to make this dairy-free.

6 pork chops, cut 1 inch thick
1 small onion, diced
2 tablespoons butter
1 apple, peeled and diced
¼ cup seedless white raisins
½ teaspoon nutmeg
¼ teaspoon cinnamon
1 cup dried egg-free bread, crumbled (see note p. 35)

Cut a pocket in each of the pork chops and pound flat. Sauté onion in butter in a skillet until golden; add apple, raisins, nutmeg, and cinnamon. Add crumbled bread, tossing well. Add several tablespoons of water, if necessary to hold mixture together. Spoon into the pocket in each pork chop and fasten edges with toothpicks. Place chops in a roasting pan in a 350° F. oven for 1-1½ hours, or until tender. Turn once during baking.

Makes 6 servings

Pork Ragout

EGG-FREE
DAIRY-FREE

This recipe would make a fine veal or lamb dish for the pork-sensitive person. Cornstarch may be used in place of flour—use half as much.

1 pound boneless pork shoulder,
   cut into 1-inch cubes
1 tablespoon salad oil
½ cup chopped onion
1 clove garlic, minced
1 carrot, pared and sliced
½ pound fresh mushrooms,
   sliced

2 tablespoons flour
2 cups chicken broth
1 teaspoon salt
⅛ teaspoon pepper
1 bay leaf
½ teaspoon dried thyme
2 cups shredded cabbage

Brown meat in salad oil in a Dutch oven. Add onion, garlic, carrot, and mushrooms. Cook 5 minutes or until vegetables are crisp-tender. Sprinkle with flour and mix well. Stir in broth. Add salt, pepper, bay leaf, and thyme. Cover and cook over low heat 1 hour. Add cabbage and cook 20 minutes longer.

Makes 4 servings

Chicken

Oven-Fried Chicken

EGG-FREE

This is the way to serve crispy chicken for those who can't have an egg-batter. Crushed cold uncooked rice cereal can be used in place of the flour and breadcrumbs in the coating.

1 fryer chicken, cut up
½ cup milk
¼ cup wheat flour
¼ cup fine egg-free breadcrumbs
   (see note on p. 35)

1 teaspoon salt
1 teaspoon paprika
¼ teaspoon pepper
¼ cup salad oil

Dip chicken parts in milk, soaking well. Combine flour, breadcrumbs, salt, paprika, and pepper; dip chicken parts into this mixture, coating heavily. Pour salad oil into a shallow baking pan and add chicken, skin side down. Bake in a 400° F. oven for 30 minutes; turn chicken and bake 30 minutes more, or until tender.

Makes 8 servings

Baked Chicken Pêche

EGG-FREE

Cornstarch and dairy-free margarine may be used in place of the flour and butter, if desired. Pecans may be omitted if there is a sensitivity to nuts.

2 fryer chickens, cut up	¼ cup orange juice
¼ cup flour	1 29-ounce can peach slices
6 tablespoons butter	½ cup pecan halves

Dredge chickens lightly in flour and shake off excess. Melt 4 tablespoons of the butter in a skillet; brown the chicken lightly. Transfer chicken parts to a baking dish. Add remaining 2 tablespoons of butter to the skillet and melt. Stir in orange juice. Stir in ¾ cup of the peach liquid. Pour mixture over the chicken. Bake in a 350° F. oven for 1 hour, basting occasionally with the liquid. Add peaches between the chicken parts and dot the top with pecans; bake 15 minutes longer, basting with remaining liquid in baking pan.

Makes 8 servings

Baked Chicken in Apricot Sauce

EGG-FREE
DAIRY-FREE

For a gluten-free recipe, prepare with cornstarch instead of wheat flour. The garlic and ginger are the taste enhancers!

2 fryer chickens, cut up	¼ cup salad oil
¼ cup wheat flour	1 8-ounce can apricot halves
1 teaspoon paprika	2 tablespoons lemon juice
½ teaspoon salt	¼ teaspoon garlic powder
¼ teaspoon pepper	¼ teaspoon ginger

Wash and dry chicken parts. Combine flour, paprika, salt, and pepper; dredge chicken parts to coat well. Heat oil in a skillet; brown chicken parts in oil. Transfer chicken to a baking dish. Pour contents of can of apricots into an electric blender; add lemon juice, garlic powder, and ginger and process into a smooth puree. Pour over the chicken. Cover with a lid or with aluminum foil. Bake in a 350° F. oven for 1 hour, or until fork tender.

Makes 8 servings

Chicken Pecan Salad

EGG-FREE
GLUTEN-FREE

When you need a creamy dressing to hold a salad together, think of plain yogurt. Flavor it with herbs to heighten piquancy.

1½ cups chopped cooked chicken
3 tablespoons chopped pecans
¼ cup diced celery
2 tablespoons grated carrot
½ cup plain yogurt
1 teaspoon chopped dillweed
¼ teaspoon salt
Dash of pepper

Combine chicken, pecans, celery, and carrot. Toss with yogurt, dillweed, salt, and pepper. Use as a salad or as a sandwich spread.

Makes 2 ½ cups.

Roast Chicken with Apple Stuffing

EGG-FREE

Why make a plain roasted chicken when, with a little effort, you can stuff it with elegance? Dairy-free margarine and bread cubes would make it safe for the milk-allergic.

3 tablespoons butter
¼ cup chopped fresh onion
½ cup chopped celery
2 tablespoons chopped nuts
2 cups chopped pared cooking apples
1 teaspoon salt
¼ teaspoon dried sage
¼ teaspoon cinnamon
1 teaspoon sugar
1 orange, sectioned
1 cup toasted egg-free bread cubes (see note on p. 35)
1 roasting chicken, about 5 pounds

Melt butter in a skillet; add onion and celery and cook until tender. Add nuts, apples, salt, sage, cinnamon, and sugar. Continue cooking until apples can be pierced with a fork but are not soft, about 10 minutes. Combine orange sections with bread cubes and apple mixture. Stuff into cavity of cleaned roasting chicken. Roast in a 350° F. oven for 1½-2 hours, or until thickest part of chicken is fork-tender.

Makes 6 servings

Nutty Fried Chicken

EGG-FREE
GLUTEN-FREE

How nutty can we get? Just switch to dairy-free margarine to make this OK for those sensitive to milk.

8 chicken legs or thighs
½ cup peanut butter
4 tablespoons butter

1½ cups finely chopped salted peanuts

Rinse and dry chicken parts. Melt peanut butter and butter together. Dip chicken parts into melted mixture and then roll in chopped peanuts. Place on a greased pan and bake in a 375° F. oven for 1 hour, or until tender.

Makes 4 servings

Chicken Livers and Grapefruit

EGG-FREE
GLUTEN-FREE

Use dairy-free margarine instead of butter to make this suitable for the dairy-sensitive. So complementary, chicken livers and grapefruit!

1 tablespoon butter
¼ cup chopped onion
2 tablespoons chopped parsley
1 pound chicken livers, halved
¼ teaspoon salt
¼ cup grapefruit juice
2 cups grapefruit sections
Hot rice (optional)

Melt butter in a large skillet. Add onion and sauté until tender. Add parsley, chicken livers, salt, and grapefruit juice. Cover and simmer over low heat for 10 minutes. Add grapefruit sections and serve on hot cooked rice.

Makes 4 servings

Fish

Baked Red Snapper in Sauce

EGG-FREE

Omit the flour altogether if there's a gluten problem. Vegetable oil may be used in place of butter.

3 pounds whole red snapper, cleaned
⅓ cup flour
½ teaspoon salt
⅛ teaspoon pepper
3 tablespoons butter
1 small onion, diced
1 cup diced celery
1 small green pepper, diced
1 clove garlic, minced
4 tomatoes, skinned and chopped
½ teaspoon chili powder
¼ cup lemon juice
2 bay leaves

Lightly dredge fish in mixture of flour, salt, and pepper. Place in a buttered baking dish. Melt butter in a skillet; sauté onion, celery, green pepper, and garlic until all are limp. Add chopped tomatoes, chili powder, and lemon juice. Pour this mixture around the fish. Add bay leaves. Bake uncovered in a 350° F. oven for 45 minutes, or until fish flakes easily. Baste occasionally with sauce.

Makes 4–6 servings

Broiled Red Snapper

EGG-FREE
GLUTEN-FREE

Lime juice plumps up the fish and gives extra flavor. Use dairy-free margarine if butter is off your list.

4 red snapper fillets
¼ cup lime juice
½ teaspoon salt

⅛ teaspoon pepper
⅛ teaspoon paprika
1 tablespoon butter

Arrange red snapper fillets in a shallow baking pan; pour lime juice over fish and let stand 10 minutes. Sprinkle with salt, pepper, and paprika. Dot with bits of butter. Broil for 8–10 minutes, or until fish flakes easily.

Makes 4 servings

Baked Flounder with Mushrooms

EGG-FREE

You can get delightful dairy-free results when fish stock replaces the milk, dairy-free margarine replaces the butter, and the cheese is omitted. Use 1 tablespoon of cornstarch as the thickener, if preferred.

4 tablespoons butter
4 flounder fillets
½ pound fresh mushrooms,
    sliced
1 tablespoon flour
1 cup milk

1 teaspoon grated onion
½ teaspoon dried dillweed
¼ teaspoon salt
⅛ teaspoon pepper
2 tablespoons grated
    Parmesan cheese

Melt 2 tablespoons of the butter in a flat baking dish. Arrange fish in a single layer. Melt remaining 2 tablespoons of butter in a saucepan; add mushrooms and sauté until limp. Remove mushrooms with a slotted spoon and spread over the fish. Add flour to the remaining butter in the saucepan; cook and stir until mixture is thick and bubbling. Remove from heat and gradually add milk until smooth. Cook again, stirring constantly, until thick. Add onion, dillweed, salt, and pepper. Spread over mushrooms on fish. Sprinkle grated Parmesan cheese over all. Bake in a preheated 350° F. oven for 25 minutes, or until fish flakes easily.

Makes 4 servings

Flounder Florentine

EGG-FREE
GLUTEN-FREE

Flounder and spinach have a fascination for each other. Dairy-free margarine makes it milk-free, if necessary.

4 slices fillet of flounder
1 10-ounce package frozen chopped spinach,
    thawed and drained
1 tablespoon grated onion
¼ teaspoon nutmeg
¼ teaspoon salt
2 tablespoons melted butter
2 tablespoons lemon juice
Paprika

Lay fillets of flounder flat on a work surface. Combine spinach, onion, nutmeg, and salt; spread in a thin layer over top surface of fillets. Roll up, fastening with toothpicks if necessary. Place in a greased baking pan. Combine melted butter and lemon juice; brush over tops of fish rolls. Sprinkle with paprika. Bake uncovered in a 350° F. oven for 20 minutes, or until fish flakes easily.

Makes 4 servings

Stuffed Flounder with Orange Sauce

EGG-FREE

This is almost a meal in itself—a salad or a vegetable completes the menu. Use 1½ teaspoons cornstarch in place of the flour and dairy-free margarine instead of butter, if desired.

1 cup cooked rice
2 tablespoons chopped
  fresh dillweed
2 tablespoons butter,
  melted
6 flounder fillets

1 tablespoon butter
1 tablespoon flour
1 cup orange juice
2 tablespoons lemon juice
1 tablespoon slivered
  almonds

Combine rice, dillweed, and melted butter. Spread a thin layer on each of the flounder fillets; roll up and place in a baking pan. Bake in a 350° F. oven for 20-25 minutes, or until fish flakes easily. Meanwhile, melt 1 tablespoon butter in a saucepan; stir in flour and cook until bubbling. Remove from heat and gradually stir in orange juice and lemon juice. Cook again, stirring constantly, until sauce thickens. Spoon sauce over cooked fish rolls. Garnish with slivered almonds and serve at once.

Makes 6 servings

Cashew Banana Sole

EGG-FREE
GLUTEN-FREE

Switch from butter to dairy-free margarine to make this milk-free. The cashews are a delectable addition.

4 large fillets of sole (about 2 pounds)
½ teaspoon salt
⅛ teaspoon pepper
4 tablespoons butter
2 bananas, sliced
2 tablespoons lemon juice
¼ cup chopped cashews

Arrange fish slices flat in a buttered baking dish. Sprinkle with salt and pepper. Dot with 3 tablespoons of the butter. Cover tightly and bake in a 350° F. oven for 20 minutes. Meanwhile, toss banana slices with lemon juice. Melt remaining tablespoon butter in a skillet. Add cashews and sliced banana; cook over low heat for several minutes. Spoon over cooked fish.

Makes 4 servings

Boiled Salmon with Dill Sauce

EGG-FREE
GLUTEN-FREE

Simmered salmon is delicious both hot and cold. Those sensitive to dairy products may skip the dill sauce.

4 small salmon steaks
Boiling water
1 lemon, sliced thin
½ teaspoon salt

Place salmon steaks on a rack in the bottom of a fish poacher or large skillet. Cover with boiling water. Add sliced lemon and salt. Simmer for about 10 minutes, or until fish flakes easily but holds its shape. Remove fish and serve hot or cold with Dill Sauce.

Makes 4 servings

Dill Sauce

1 cup plain yogurt
2 tablespoons chopped chives
1 tablespoon lemon juice
½ teaspoon salt
1 tablespoon minced fresh dill

Empty yogurt into a bowl. Stir in chives. Add lemon juice, salt, and dill.

Makes 1 cup

Stuffed Bluefish

EGG-FREE

For gluten-allergies, use wheat-free cornbread in the stuffing.

Use dairy-free margarine to replace butter and tomato juice in place of milk if there is a dairy sensitivity.

2 tablespoons butter
1 small onion, diced
1 cup egg-free breadcrumbs
   (see note on p. 35)
1 teaspoon finely chopped
   parsley

½ cup chopped celery
½ teaspoon salt
¼ cup milk
1 whole bluefish, about
   4 pounds, cleaned
1 lemon

Melt butter in a skillet: sauté onion until tender. Stir into breadcrumbs; add celery, parsley, and salt. Stir in milk. Wash and wipe bluefish: stuff with prepared mixture. Cut lemon in half and squeeze over fish. Place in a greased pan. Bake for 15 minutes per pound of fish in a 375° F. oven.

Makes 4 servings

Curried Shrimp

EGG-FREE
GLUTEN-FREE

The apple and curry give the shrimp a tasty kick. Those with dairy allergies can use oil in place of butter.

4 tablespoons butter
1 onion, diced fine
1 green pepper, diced fine
1 small apple, peeled, cored,
   and chopped fine
½ teaspoon salt

⅛ teaspoon pepper
1 teaspoon curry powder
1 1-pound can tomatoes
1 pound raw shrimp,
   cleaned and peeled

Melt butter in a skillet; add onion, green pepper, apple, salt, pepper, and curry powder. Stir and cook until onion is limp. Add tomatoes, breaking them up with a fork as they cook. Add shrimp. Cover and simmer for 10–15 minutes, or until shrimp are cooked through.

Makes 4 servings

Halibut au Gratin

EGG-FREE

The breadcrumbs can be omitted for gluten-sensitivities. Dairy-allergic people should use water in place of cream, omit the cheese, and use dairy-free margarine to dot the fish. It will still have a lovely flavor!

1 onion
½ pound fresh mushrooms
2 tablespoons minced parsley
4 halibut steaks
¼ cup lemon juice
½ teaspoon salt
⅛ teaspoon pepper
½ cup light cream

¼ cup fine egg-free breadcrumbs, (see note on p. 35)
2 tablespoons grated hard white cheese
4 teaspoons butter
4 lemon wedges

Chop onion, mushrooms, and parsley together; place in a thin layer over the bottom of a buttered baking dish. Arrange fish on top. Sprinkle with lemon juice, salt, and pepper. Pour cream around fish. Sprinkle breadcrumbs and cheese over fish and dot with butter. Bake in a 375° F. oven for 3 minutes. Serve with lemon wedges.

Makes 4 servings

Oyster Stew

EGG-FREE
GLUTEN-FREE

Have the fish seller shuck the oysters for you and this will be an easy dish to make. Don't overcook or the oysters will be tough!

1 pint shucked oysters, with liquid
1 quart milk
¼ cup butter

1 sprig fresh dillweed
½ teaspoon salt
⅛ teaspoon pepper

In a 2-quart saucepan, cook oysters, with liquid, over low heat until edges of oysters just begin to curl. Add milk, butter, dillweed, salt, and pepper. Heat slowly until hot; do not boil.

Makes about 6 servings

Scalloped Oysters

EGG-FREE

Here's another way to prepare oysters—let the oven bake them to perfection. Those allergic to milk and wheat will have to pass this one by.

1 quart shucked oysters, with liquid
2 cups coarsely crushed soda crackers
½ cup butter
1–2 cups milk
1 tablespoon chopped parsley
½ teaspoon salt
⅛ teaspoon pepper

In a greased 2-quart casserole, alternate layers of oysters with layers of liquid and crackers, dotting each layer with butter and sprinkling with parsley, salt, and pepper. End with a layer of crackers. Add milk until the liquid almost reaches the top of the casserole. Dot with the remaining butter. Bake in a 350° F. oven until browned, 45–60 minutes.

Makes 6–8 servings

Mussels Provençal

EGG-FREE
GLUTEN-FREE

Here's the easiest and possibly the best way to enjoy mussels. Memories of Moules Provençal in Brussels prompt this frank imitation!

1 pound fresh mussels in the shell
2 shallots or 4 green onions, chopped
1 cup white wine
4 tablespoons butter
½ teaspoon thyme
½ teaspoon rosemary
2 teaspoons chopped parsley
⅛ teaspoon pepper

Scrub and clean mussels thoroughly just before cooking, changing the water several times until it is completely clear. Put mussels in a large deep pot with shallots or onions, wine, 1 tablespoon of the butter, thyme, rosemary, parsley, and pepper. Bring to a fast boil, shaking the pot as the mussels open. Transfer mussels to a serving bowl. Cook liquid until reduced to half of its original volume. Add the remaining butter and stir until it is melted. Pour over the mussels and serve hot.

Makes 4 servings

Tuna Roesti

EGG-FREE
GLUTEN-FREE

Good old tuna takes on an air of serious dining when tucked into this baked potato creation.

3 cups sliced cooked
  potatoes
¼ cup chopped onion
2 7-ounce cans tuna,
  drained and flaked

½ teaspoon salt
1 cup grated Gruyère
  cheese
¼ cup butter

Combine potato slices, chopped onion, tuna, salt, and grated cheese. Melt butter in a large skillet. Add tuna mixture and press firmly over bottom of the skillet. Cook over medium heat until a golden brown crust forms on the bottom. Turn mixture with a spatula, in several sections if necessary, and brown other side.

Makes 4–6 servings

Tuna Cauliflower Casserole

EGG-FREE

If all butter is replaced with dairy-free margarine, and tomato juice is used in place of milk, this becomes fare for milk-allergy sufferers. To make it gluten-free, thicken with 1 tablespoon of cornstarch instead of the flour and skip the breadcrumbs.

1 small head cauliflower, cut into small flowerets
½ cup boiling water
1 teaspoon salt
2 tablespoons butter
2 tablespoons flour
1⅓ cups milk
⅛ teaspoon minced garlic
⅛ teaspoon thyme
⅛ teaspoon white pepper
1 7-ounce can tuna, drained and flaked
1 tablespoon butter, melted
½ cup soft egg-free breadcrumbs (see note on page 35)

Place cauliflower, boiling water, and salt in a saucepan. Bring to the boiling point, uncovered; cover and boil 3 minutes, or until partly done. Drain and set aside. Melt 2 tablespoons butter in a saucepan; blend in flour. Remove from heat and gradually stir in milk. Stir and cook over medium heat until thick. Remove from heat and add garlic, thyme, and pepper. Add cauliflower and tuna, spoon into a buttered 1-quart casserole. Combine 1 tablespoon melted butter and breadcrumbs; sprinkle over the top. Bake in a 350° F. oven for 35 minutes, or until golden brown.

Makes 6 servings

VEGETABLES

Baked Acorn Squash

EGG-FREE
GLUTEN-FREE

Using dairy-free margarine makes this milk-free. So surprising to find a vegetable that can please a sweet tooth!

2 acorn squash
2 teaspoons honey
1 teaspoon butter
¼ teaspoon salt
¼ teaspoon cinnamon

Preheat oven to 350° F. Cut acorn squash in half lengthwise. Scoop out and discard seeds. Place squash, cut side up, in a baking pan. Fill cavities with honey. Dot with butter. Sprinkle with salt and cinnamon. Bake in a 350° F. oven for 25–30 minutes, or until fork-tender.

Makes 4 servings

Cole Slaw with Yogurt Dressing

EGG-FREE
GLUTEN-FREE

This has a creamy dressing that is thickened and sweetened with a bit of honey. Celery seed gives an extra kick of flavor.

1 cup plain yogurt
2 teaspoons vinegar
2 teaspoons honey
1 tablespoon grated onion
1 teaspoon celery seed

¼ teaspoon salt
⅛ teaspoon pepper
⅛ teaspoon dry mustard
2 cups shredded cabbage

Combine yogurt, vinegar, and honey; mix until smoothly blended. Add onion, celery seed, salt, pepper, and mustard. Toss with cabbage. Chill.

Makes 4 servings

Green Beans in Cheddar Sauce

EGG-FREE

Green beans can be steamed and served crispy and brimming with vitamins. The delicious cheddar sauce is for those who can tolerate milk products. It can be made gluten-free by using 1½ teaspoons of cornstarch instead of the flour.

1 pound fresh green beans
1 tablespoon butter
1 tablespoon flour
1 cup milk
¼ cup grated white cheddar cheese
½ teaspoon salt
⅛ teaspoon pepper

Trim and wash green beans. Place in a saucepan and cover with water; bring to a boil and then simmer for 5 minutes, or until tender. (If preferred, steam beans over boiling water.) Meanwhile, melt butter in a saucepan; stir in flour until bubbling. Remove from heat and gradually stir in milk. Return to heat and cook until thickened, stirring constantly. Add grated cheese, salt, and pepper; stir until cheese is well blended. Toss cooked beans with this sauce and serve.

Makes 4 servings

Green Beans and Mushrooms

EGG-FREE
GLUTEN-FREE

Using dairy-free margarine instead of butter makes this a dish for the milk-sensitive. The soy sauce adds a fascinating flavor.

2 10-ounce packages frozen cut green beans, or 1 pound fresh fresh green beans
½ cup fresh sliced mushrooms
2 tablespoons butter
½ teaspoon pure soy sauce

Steam fresh green beans or cook frozen green beans as directed on the package. Drain. Sauté mushrooms in butter; add green beans. Add soy sauce and toss lightly.

Makes 6 servings

Broccoli with Mushroom Sauce

EGG-FREE
GLUTEN-FREE

Pick tight-budded broccoli heads and don't overcook! Use dairy-free margarine in place of butter, if desired.

1 large bunch broccoli
½ teaspoon salt
2 tablespoons butter

½ cup chopped fresh mushrooms
1 teaspoon lemon juice

Trim broccoli of excess leaves and rough stems. Scrape with a vegetable peeler to remove thin outer layer. (This permits the broccoli to become tender more quickly.) Place in a heavy saucepan and cover with water. Add salt and cook for 15 minutes, or until fork-tender. Melt butter in a small skillet; sauté mushrooms until limp. Stir in lemon juice and pour all over drained broccoli on a platter. Serve at once.

Makes 4–6 servings

Lemon-Buttered Cabbage

EGG-FREE
GLUTEN-FREE

Dairy-free margarine can replace butter to make this cabbage dish milk-free.

¼ cup butter
1 large head cabbage,
  shredded
½ teaspoon grated lemon
  peel

2 tablespoons lemon juice
½ teaspoon celery seed
½ teaspoon salt
⅛ teaspoon pepper

Melt butter in a large skillet. Add shredded cabbage. Cover and cook, stirring occasionally, about 6–8 minutes, or until just tender. Add lemon peel, lemon juice, celery seed, salt, and pepper. Serve at once.

Makes 6 servings

Hot Apple Slaw

EGG-FREE
GLUTEN-FREE

Who says that coleslaw has to be chilled? Here it is hot and tangy and ever so good. Substitute dairy-free margarine for butter for the milk-sensitive diner.

3 cups shredded cabbage
2 tablespoons cider vinegar
2 teaspoons brown sugar
2 tablespoons butter

1 teaspoon dried tarragon
¼ teaspoon salt
2 cups grated raw apples

Place cabbage in a saucepan with vinegar, brown sugar, butter, tarragon, and salt. Bring to the boiling point. Stir in apples, reduce heat, and cook for several minutes until apples are hot. Serve hot.

Makes 4 servings

Carrots Tarragon

EGG-FREE
GLUTEN-FREE

Why let carrots become dull fare, when you can pep them up with a few dashes of tarragon! Dairy-free margarine is the substitute for butter to make this milk-free.

1 pound slender fresh carrots
1 cup water
1 teaspoon dried leaf tarragon
½ teaspoon salt
2 tablespoons butter

Scrape carrots and cut into ¼-inch crosswise slices. Place in a saucepan with water, tarragon, and salt. Cover and cook over medium heat about 20 minutes or until tender. Drain, add butter, and toss.

Makes 6 servings

Baked Whole Cauliflower

EGG-FREE

There's no sense breaking up a good thing—keep the cauliflower whole during cooking. The sauce will appeal to all. Gluten-sensitive diners should exchange 1 tablespoon cornstarch for the flour and eliminate the breadcrumbs. Those allergic to dairy products can use tomato juice in place of the milk, dairy-free margarine instead of the butter, and skip the grated cheese.

**1 head cauliflower, washed
  and trimmed**
Water
½ teaspoon salt
2 tablespoons butter
2 tablespoons flour
1 cup milk
¼ teaspoon salt
⅛ teaspoon pepper
**3 tablespoons fine egg-free
  breadcrumbs
    (see note on page 35)**
**1 tablespoon grated
  Parmesan cheese**

Place cauliflower in a deep saucepan, cover with water, and add the ½ teaspoon salt. Boil for 20 minutes, or until tender but not falling apart. Drain. Place whole in a buttered baking dish. Melt butter in a saucepan and add flour, stirring constantly until blended and thick. Remove from heat and gradually stir in milk, salt, and pepper, until mixture is smooth. Return to heat, stirring constantly, until mixture is thick and bubbling. Pour evenly over the prepared cauliflower. Sprinkle bread-crumbs and Parmesan cheese over top. Place in a 375° F. oven and bake for 15–20 minutes, or until lightly browned.

Makes 6 servings

Broccoli with Cheese Sauce

EGG-FREE

This is definitely a dairy lover's dream vegetable dish! Exchange 1 tablespoon of cornstarch for flour if there's a gluten problem.

4 stalks fresh broccoli	**2 tablespoons flour**
(about 1 pound)	**¼ teaspoon salt**
2 cups water	**⅛ teaspoon pepper**
½ teaspoon salt	**1 cup milk**
2 tablespoons butter	**½ cup diced Swiss cheese**

Wash broccoli stalks well. With a vegetable parer, scrape off the outer layer of the stalks (this will produce more tender broccoli in less cooking time). Cut each stalk lengthwise into quarters. Place in a saucepan with water and the ½ teaspoon salt; cook broccoli about 12 minutes, or until tender. Meanwhile, melt butter in a saucepan; blend in flour, the ¼ teaspoon salt, and pepper. Stir constantly until smooth; then gradually stir in milk. Cook and stir until mixture boils; add cheese and stir until melted. Remove broccoli from water and drain; serve with cheese sauce.

Makes 4 servings

Orange-Glazed Beets

EGG-FREE

Whoever doesn't eat beets in your house may have a change of mind with this sweet way to indulge. Substitute dairy-free margarine for butter or 1 teaspoon cornstarch for the flour, if substitutions are in order.

1 1-pound can whole beets
1 tablespoon butter
2 teaspoons flour
1 teaspoon honey
½ cup orange juice

Heat beets in their own liquid. Melt butter in a small saucepan; stir in flour until smooth. Remove from heat. Add honey and orange juice; stir until smooth. Return to heat, stirring constantly, until thickened. Drain hot beets; pour sauce over them and serve.

Makes 4 servings

Cauliflower with Parsley Sauce

EGG-FREE

Use 1 teaspoon cornstarch in place of flour, if desired.

1 medium cauliflower   **1½ teaspoons salt**
Boiling water   **Fresh Parsley Sauce (below)**

Remove outer leaves from cauliflower, leaving small tender leaves attached. Wash thoroughly. Place whole head in a saucepan with 1 inch of boiling water and salt. Bring to boiling point without cover. Cook 5 minutes. Cover and cook 15 minutes, or until cauliflower is tender. Remove from saucepan and place in a serving dish. Top with Fresh Parsley Sauce.

Makes 6 servings

Fresh Parsley Sauce

1½ tablespoons butter
1½ tablespoons flour
1 cup hot chicken broth
½ cup light cream

1½ teaspoons salt
⅛ teaspoon pepper
⅓ cup chopped fresh parsley

Melt butter in a saucepan. Blend in flour. Remove from heat and stir in broth. Cook, stirring, until mixture begins to thicken. Add cream, salt, pepper, and parsley. Cook until medium-thick.

Makes about 1½ cups

Hot Herbed Cucumbers

EGG-FREE
GLUTEN-FREE

Cooked cucumbers? What will they think of next? Use dairy-free margarine if you must.

2 medium cucumbers, pared and sliced
1 teaspoon salt
¼ cup butter
½ teaspoon dried tarragon

Sprinkle sliced cucumbers with salt and let stand for 30 minutes. Drain well. Melt butter in a saucepan. Add drained cucumbers and tarragon. Cover and cook for 10 minutes.

Makes 6 servings

Peas in Cheese Sauce

EGG-FREE

Here's a way to dress up an ordinary vegetable like peas. The same sauce may be used for green beans.

2 10-ounce packages frozen peas
1 tablespoon butter
1 tablespoon flour
¼ teaspoon salt
⅛ teaspoon dry mustard
½ cup milk
½ cup grated Swiss cheese
½ cup diced cheddar cheese

Cook peas as directed on package. Drain. Melt butter in a large saucepan. Blend in flour, salt, and mustard. Stir in milk and cook over medium heat, stirring until thickened. Add cheese; heat until melted. Gently stir in peas and heat through.

Makes 8 servings

Peas and Water Chestnuts

EGG-FREE
GLUTEN-FREE

Exchange dairy-free margarine for butter, if desired. Don't miss this crunchy way to serve common peas.

2 pounds fresh or 2 10-ounce packages frozen peas
1 tablespoon butter
1 5-ounce can water chestnuts, drained and sliced
¼ teaspoon salt
¼ teaspoon nutmeg

Cook peas in water until tender, or steam them if preferred. Drain. Toss with butter, sliced water chestnuts, salt, and nutmeg. Serve at once.

Makes 8 servings

Scalloped Potatoes

EGG-FREE

You can thicken these scalloped potatoes with 2 tablespoons of cornstarch instead of flour if there is a sensitivity to gluten.

4 cups sliced peeled raw potatoes (¼ inch thick)
4 tablespoons flour
1 teaspoon salt
¼ teaspoon pepper
2 tablespoons butter
2 cups milk

Arrange potato slices in layers in a buttered baking dish; sprinkle each layer with combined flour, salt, and pepper. Dot each layer with bits of butter. Pour milk over top and bake in a 350° F. oven for 40 minutes, or until potatoes are tender.

Makes 6 servings

Potatoes Anna

EGG-FREE
GLUTEN-FREE

Here's a simple layered look for the mighty good potato. Use dairy-free margarine in place of butter, if you wish.

4 large baking potatoes   **1 teaspoon salt**
¼ cup melted butter   **¼ teaspoon pepper**

Peel potatoes and slice thin; soak in salted water for 30 minutes. Butter a 9-inch pie pan. Drain potatoes. Arrange a layer of potatoes in it, brush with melted butter, and sprinkle with salt and pepper. Continue to layer the potatoes, brushing with butter and sprinkling with salt and pepper, until all ingredients are used. Bake in a 400° F. oven for 35 minutes, or until potatoes are fork-tender and top is crusty.

Makes 4–6 servings

Creamed Spinach

EGG-FREE

You can thicken the cream sauce by using 1 tablespoon of cornstarch in place of the flour. Those allergic to milk products can add the onion and nutmeg to the spinach and omit the sauce.

2 10-ounce packages frozen chopped spinach
1 teaspoon grated onion
¼ teaspoon ground nutmeg
2 tablespoons butter
2 tablespoons flour
1 cup milk
½ teaspoon salt
⅛ teaspoon pepper

Place frozen spinach, grated onion, and nutmeg in a saucepan. Cover with water, cover saucepan, and cook for 10 minutes, or until tender. Drain well. Melt butter in a saucepan, stir in flour, and cook until bubbling. Remove from heat and stir in milk, salt, and pepper until smooth. Cook again, stirring constantly, until mixture thickens. Pour over drained spinach and mix well.

Makes 6 servings

Broiled Tomatoes

EGG-FREE
GLUTEN-FREE

Don't let these tomatoes get soft and soggy by overcooking. Just a bit of broiling makes them hot and yet firm.

6 tomatoes
¼ teaspoon salt
¼ teaspoon oregano
2 tablespoons grated Parmesan cheese
1 tablespoon butter

Wash tomatoes and cut in half. Arrange tomatoes, cut sides up, in a shallow baking dish. Sprinkle tops with salt, oregano, and cheese. Dot with butter. Broil for about 8 minutes or until topping is browned but tomatoes still hold shape.

Makes 6 servings

Herbed Zucchini

EGG-FREE
GLUTEN-FREE

Here is zucchini, herbed and simply delicious. Use dairy-free margarine instead of butter, if desired.

2 pounds zucchini
1 teaspoon salt
¼ teaspoon thyme
2 tablespoons butter, melted
2 tablespoons lemon juice

Wash zucchini and trim off ends. Slice zucchini into ¼-inch circles. Place in a large skillet and cover with water. Add salt and thyme. Bring to a boil, cover, and reduce heat to a simmer. Cook about 5 minutes, or until just tender. Drain. Combine melted butter and lemon juice; pour over zucchini and serve.

Makes 6 servings

PASTA AND PASTA SAUCES

Egg-Free Pasta

EGG-FREE
DAIRY-FREE

When purchasing pasta, be sure to read the label on the pasta package. Most commercial pasta is made with oil and without eggs, except for noodles. When you make your own, you can be sure!

3 cups unbleached flour or semolina flour, sifted
¾ teaspoon salt
2 tablespoons olive oil, or other salad oil
¾ cup warm water

Make a well in the center of the sifted flour. Add salt, olive oil, and ¼ cup of the water. Knead this mixture together, adding more water as necessary to form a soft dough. When dough feels smooth, cover it with a bowl or clean kitchen towel and allow it to rest for at least 10 minutes. Reknead the dough until it seems to have an elastic quality and is quite smooth. Cover again for 10 minutes. Divide the dough into four parts; roll each part thin (or process through a hand or electric pasta roller) and cut into the width desired. Spread on clean towels or hang on a doweled pasta rack to dry for one hour. Cook in boiling salted water for 5 to 8 minutes (homemade pasta takes less time to cook than commercial pasta—test the strands frequently during cooking to be sure not to overcook). Serve with Pesto Sauce, Alfredo Sauce, or preferred sauce.

Makes 1 pound

Alfredo Sauce

EGG-FREE
GLUTEN-FREE

Homemade pasta is delicious with a simple cream, butter, and cheese sauce, as served in the famous Alfredo's restaurant in Rome. Here is a reasonable facsimile to make at home.

2 tablespoons butter	**¼ teaspoon salt**
¾ cup heavy cream	**⅛ teaspoon pepper**
½ cup grated Parmesan cheese	**⅛ teaspoon nutmeg**

Melt butter in a saucepan. Add cream and cook over low heat. Add half of the grated cheese, salt, pepper, and nutmeg. Cook and stir for a minute. Pour over cooked pasta, top with remaining grated cheese, and serve at once.

Makes about 1 cup

Pesto Sauce

EGG-FREE/
GLUTEN-FREE

Fresh basil leaves are available in the summer—you might even grow a good supply in your garden. If you think ahead and freeze one cup of leaves in each of many small self-lock plastic bags, you will have an ample supply for the rest of the year.

1 cup fresh basil leaves
2 tablespoons shelled pignoli nuts (pine nuts)
2 cloves fresh garlic, finely minced
¼ cup olive oil
2 tablespoons grated Parmesan cheese
¼ teaspoon salt
⅛ teaspoon pepper

Wash basil leaves well; remove the stems. Place in a blender or food processor with remaining ingredients. Process into a smooth green sauce. Pour over hot drained pasta and serve.

Makes about 1 cup

NOTE: Sauce may be made in larger quantities and frozen in ice cube trays. Remove Pesto cubes to a plastic bag and freeze until needed. Just heat to use.

BREADS AND GRAINS

Egg-Free White Bread

EGG-FREE

This white bread becomes dairy-free when the butter is replaced by dairy-free margarine. Bake one for today and one for the freezer!

7¾–8¾ cups unsifted flour
3 tablespoons sugar
½ teaspoon salt
3 packages active dry yeast
⅓ cup butter
2⅔ cups very warm water (about 110°F.)
Peanut oil

In a large bowl, thoroughly mix 3 cups of the flour, the sugar, salt, and undissolved yeast. Add the butter. Gradually add the warm water to the dry ingredients and beat with an electric mixer for 2 minutes at medium speed, scraping the bowl occasionally. Add ½ cup flour. Beat at high speed for 2 minutes, occasionally scraping the bowl. Stir in enough additional flour to make a stiff dough. Turn out onto a lightly floured breadboard; knead until smooth and elastic (about 10–12 minutes). Cover with plastic wrap, then a towel. Let rest 20 minutes. Divide dough in half. Roll each half into a 9-by-14-inch rectangle. Shape into loaves by rolling the upper short side toward you. Seal with thumbs. Seal ends; fold sealed ends under. Be careful not to tear the dough.

Grease two 9-by-5-by-3-inch loaf pans with butter. Place the loaves in the pans, seam side down. Brush with peanut oil. Cover loosely with plastic wrap. Refrigerate 2–24 hours. When ready to bake, remove from refrigerator and uncover dough carefully. Let stand at room temperature 10 minutes. Puncture any gas bubbles that may have formed, using a greased toothpick or metal skewer. Bake in a 400° F. oven for 35–40 minutes, or until done. Remove from baking pans and cool on wire racks. Loaves may be frozen for future use.

Makes 2 loaves

Peanut Butter Yeast Bread

EGG-FREE

The peanut butter gives just a hint of flavor that makes this a very special egg-free bread.

1 cup milk
2 tablespoons sugar
2 teaspoons salt
3 tablespoons corn oil
1 cup warm water
1 package active dry yeast or 1 cake compressed yeast
About 6 cups sifted flour
½ cup creamy or chunky peanut butter
2 tablespoons melted butter

Scald milk, then stir in sugar, salt, and corn oil. Cool to lukewarm. Measure water into a warm mixing bowl. Sprinkle or crumble in yeast and stir until dissolved. Blend in lukewarm milk mixture. Add 3 cups of the flour; beat until smooth. Add remaining flour or enough to make an easily handled dough. Turn the dough out into a lightly floured board or cloth. Let rest 15 minutes. Knead until smooth and elastic. Place in an oiled bowl, smooth side down. Then turn the ball of dough so the smooth side is up. (This lightly greases the top.) Cover with a clean towel. Let rise in a warm place, free from drafts, until doubled in bulk, about 1 hour and 20 minutes. Punch down. Roll out on lightly floured board to 12-inch square. Spread with peanut butter. Roll up. Pinch dough to seal edges. Bring ends together and overlap side by side about one inch, forming a ring. Tuck inside and into center; seal. Tuck the outside end under the ring from the outside. Place on an ungreased cookie sheet. Cover; let rise as directed above until doubled in bulk, about 45 minutes. Brush with melted butter. Score the top with a knife, making 1½-inch squares. Bake in 400° F. oven until brown and crusty, about 40 minutes.

Makes 1 large loaf

Irish Soda Bread

EGG-FREE

Here's an easy no-yeast way to make a quick bread. The buttermilk adds extra good taste.

2 cups all-purpose flour	**1 teaspoon salt**
1½ teaspoons baking powder	**3 tablespoons sugar**
¼ teaspoon baking soda	**1 cup buttermilk**

Mix flour, baking powder, baking soda, salt, and sugar together. Stir in buttermilk to make a soft dough. Knead the dough on a lightly floured board for about a minute; then shape it into a round loaf and put it into an 8-inch greased round pan. Pat flour lightly over the top surface, then cut crosswise into the top. Bake in a preheated 350° F. oven for 40 minutes, or until done. Bread should have a hollow sound when tapped.

Makes 8 servings

Egg-Free Banana Bread

EGG-FREE

Bananas somehow make egg-free baked goods better. The molasses gives an old-fashioned flavor. Spread bread with cream cheese for a total triumph.

2 cups whole wheat flour	**1 cup mashed bananas**
1 cup yellow cornmeal	**1 cup buttermilk**
¾ teaspoon salt	**¾ cup unsulphured molasses**
1 teaspoon baking soda	**¾ cup raisins**

In a large bowl, mix together flour, cornmeal, salt, and baking soda. Stir in mashed bananas, buttermilk, molasses, and raisins. Turn into 3 greased and floured 1-pound cans (from canned fruit or vegetables). Bake in a preheated 350° F. oven for 45 minutes. Cool for 10 minutes, turn out of cans, and serve warm.

Makes 3 loaves

NOTE: Loaves may be frozen. Thaw and reheat in a 350° F. oven, wrapped in foil, for about 20 minutes.

Egg-Free Whole Wheat Bread

EGG-FREE

Once you have baked with yeast dough and felt its springiness as you knead it into elasticity, you'll never feel yeast-shy again. This one becomes milk-free when you exchange dairy-free margarine for the butter.

1 package active dry yeast
2¼ cups warm water
1 teaspoon sugar
2½ cups flour
3 tablespoons butter, melted
2 tablespoons molasses
1½ teaspoons salt
2 cups whole wheat flour
1 cup wheat flour

Dissolve yeast in water; add sugar and 2½ cups wheat flour. Mix well and let rise until bubbly, about 20 minutes. Add butter, molasses, salt, and whole wheat flour; beat well. Knead in just enough of the additional wheat flour to make a soft dough. Knead dough until it is smooth and elastic. Let rise in a lightly greased bowl until dough doubles in bulk. Punch down; divide in two and roll each piece to fit into two lightly greased 8½-by-4½-inch loaf pans. Allow to rise again. Bake in a 375° F. oven for 40 minutes, or until bread sounds hollow when tapped. Turn loaves out onto a wire rack to cool.

Makes 2 loaves

Drop Biscuits

EGG-FREE

When the egg-sensitive wants a quick biscuit, here's the one to make. The whole family will love it.

2 cups sifted flour   ½ cup corn oil
1 tablespoon baking powder   ¾ cup milk
1 teaspoon salt

Sift together flour, baking powder, and salt. Blend in corn oil with a fork. Add milk and mix until dough forms. Drop dough by spoonfuls onto an ungreased cookie sheet. Bake in a 450° F. oven for 12–15 minutes, or until lightly browned.

Makes 12 biscuits

Buttermilk Biscuits

EGG-FREE

If you like soft-edged biscuits, place them close together on the cookie sheet. If you prefer them crusty, place them farther apart.

2 cups sifted flour
1 tablespoon baking powder
1 teaspoon salt
¼ teaspoon baking soda
⅓ cup salad oil
⅔ cup buttermilk

Stir together flour, baking powder, salt, and baking soda. Blend in oil with a fork. Stir in buttermilk; mix until dough forms into a ball. Gently knead dough on a lightly floured board. Roll or pat out to a ½-inch thickness. Cut with a floured biscuit cutter or the floured rim of a glass and place on an ungreased cookie sheet. Bake in a preheated 450° F. oven for 12–15 minutes, or until lightly browned.

Makes 12 biscuits

Biscuits

EGG-FREE

When you have the time to roll out the biscuits and cut them into rounds, this egg-free recipe will provide a delicious reward.

2 cups sifted flour
3 teaspoons baking powder
1 teaspoon salt
4 tablespoons butter
⅔ cup milk

Sift flour, baking powder, and salt together. Cut in butter. Add milk to make a soft dough. Turn out on a floured board and knead for 30 seconds. Then roll out to a ½-inch thickness and cut with a floured biscuit cutter. Bake on an ungreased baking sheet in a 450° F. oven for 10–12 minutes.

Makes 1 dozen

Buttermilk Bran Bread

EGG-FREE

Bran adds fiber to the diet and buttermilk adds extra flavor. This makes a tasty egg-free loaf.

1⅔ cups crushed whole-bran cereal
4⅓ cups sifted flour
1 tablespoon baking soda
1 teaspoon sugar
1 teaspoon salt
2½ cups buttermilk

Preheat oven to 350° F. Mix together bran, flour, baking soda, sugar, and salt. Make a well in the center and pour in buttermilk. Work quickly and knead dough lightly; shape into a loaf and press into a greased 9-by-5-inch loaf pan in a 350° F. oven for 1 hour, or until firm and lightly browned.

Makes 1 loaf

Breakfast Rice and Raisins

EGG-FREE
GLUTEN-FREE

Why not have regular hot cooked rice for breakfast with the punch of raisins for protein and potassium? Milk-sensitive eaters can use dairy-free margarine in place of the cream and still enjoy a mighty fine morning.

2 cups hot cooked rice
2 tablespoons heavy cream
¼ cup raisins
1 teaspoon brown sugar
⅛ teaspoon cinnamon
Dash of nutmeg

While rice is cooking, combine cream, raisins, sugar, cinnamon, and nutmeg in a saucepan; bring to a boil. Stir in rice and fluff with a fork. Pour into cereal dishes.

Makes 3 servings

DESSERTS

Strawberry Banana Split

EGG-FREE
GLUTEN-FREE

Fresh berries blended with yogurt make a sauce that's nicely low in calories while tasting sinfully delicious!

2 bananas
1 pint fresh strawberries, chilled
1 cup plain yogurt
½ teaspoon pure vanilla extract

Peel and cut bananas in half lengthwise. Wash and drain

strawberries, discarding any that are overripe or underripe. Arrange each long strip of banana in the bottom of a banana split dish or cut in half and place along the rim of a dessert plate. Fill the middle of each of four plates with strawberries, reserving ½ cup of the softer berries. Place the soft berries in an electric blender with the yogurt and vanilla; blend until smooth. Pour over the arranged strawberries. Place one berry on top of each mound.

Makes 4 servings

Blanc Mange

EGG-FREE
GLUTEN-FREE

When you want a pudding despite an allergy to eggs, here's the way to concoct a reasonable facsimile.

½ cup sugar
5 tablespoons cornstarch
¼ teaspoon salt
4 cups milk
1½ teaspoons vanilla extract

Mix sugar, cornstarch, and salt in the top of a double boiler. Gradually add milk, stirring until smooth. Cook over boiling water, stirring constantly, until mixture thickens enough to mound slightly when dropped from a spoon. Cover and continue cooking 10 minutes longer, stirring occasionally. Remove from heat. Stir in vanilla. Pour into serving dish or individual dishes. Chill. Serve plain or with fresh fruit, jelly, or jam.

Makes 8 servings

Vanilla Pudding

EGG-FREE
GLUTEN-FREE

Add some fresh cut-up fruit or dried raisins to this pudding before chilling, and you'll have a dessert that is egg-free and mouthwatering.

⅓ cup sugar
¼ cup cornstarch
⅛ teaspoon salt
2¾ cups milk

2 tablespoons butter
1 teaspoon pure vanilla
   extract

Combine sugar, cornstarch, salt, and milk in a large saucepan; mix until smooth. Cook over medium heat, stirring constantly, until mixture comes to a boil; boil 1 minute and remove from heat. Stir in butter and vanilla and pour into individual serving dishes. Chill.

Makes 6 servings

Chocolate-Banana Pudding

EGG-FREE
GLUTEN-FREE

Here's another way to make a pudding without eggs. Be sure that the cocoa is the old-fashioned type and not a sugar-added mix.

2 envelopes unflavored gelatin
½ cup cold water
1 cup boiling water
¼ cup sugar
2 tablespoons unsweetened cocoa
⅔ cup nonfat dry milk powder
2 ripe bananas, cut into pieces
1 teaspoon pure vanilla extract
12 ice cubes

Sprinkle gelatin over cold water in a blender container. Add boiling water; cover and blend on low speed until gelatin is dissolved. Add sugar, cocoa, and dry milk; cover and blend until smooth. Add bananas and vanilla; blend on high speed. While blender is running, add ice cubes, one at a time. Continue blending until ice is dissolved. Quickly pour mixture into dessert dishes. Chill 20–30 minutes or until set.

Makes 8 servings

Peanut Butter Pudding

EGG-FREE
GLUTEN-FREE

If a smooth pudding is desired, use smooth peanut butter instead of the chunky kind. Either way, mighty good to eat!

½ cup brown sugar
¼ cup cornstarch
⅛ teaspoon salt
3¼ cups skim milk
¾ cup chunky peanut butter
1 teaspoon vanilla

In a 2-quart saucepan, stir together sugar, cornstarch, and salt. Gradually stir in milk until smooth. Stirring constantly, place over heat and bring to a boil; boil for one minute. Remove from heat. Stir in peanut butter and vanilla. Pour into 6 dessert dishes.

Makes 6 ½-cup servings

Variation: Chocolate Pudding

To the Peanut Butter Pudding recipe above, add 3 tablespoons unsweetened cocoa with the sugar, cornstarch, and salt.

Lacey Wafers

EGG-FREE

If you want to roll these into a cone shape, do so immediately after removal from the oven. Use vegetable shortening to make it dairy-free.

1 cup sifted wheat flour
1 cup chopped flaked coconut
½ cup light corn syrup
½ cup firmly packed brown
  sugar

½ cup butter or vegetable
  shortening
1 teaspoon pure vanilla
  extract

Mix sifted flour and coconut. Combine corn syrup, brown sugar, and butter in a heavy saucepan. Bring to a boil over medium heat, stirring constantly. Remove from heat. Gradually blend in flour-coconut mixture, then stir in vanilla. Drop by heaping tablespoonfuls onto a foil-covered cookie sheet. Bake in a 350° F. oven for 8–10 minutes. Cool on a wire rack until foil may be peeled off easily, 3–4 minutes. Cool completely on absorbent paper.

Makes about 2 dozen

Peanut Butter Chocolate Cake

EGG-FREE

If there's no allergy to chocolate, here's a reason to rejoice — egg-free chocolate cake with a kick of peanut flavor.

1¾ cups unsifted cake flour
1 cup sugar
¾ teaspoon salt
¾ teaspoon baking soda
¼ cup creamy or chunky peanut butter
2 tablespoons butter
2 1-ounce unsweetened chocolate squares, melted
1 teaspoon pure vanilla extract
1 cup buttermilk or sour milk (see following note)

Grease 2 8-by-1½-inch layer cake pans; line bottoms with waxed paper. Sift together flour, sugar, salt, and baking soda. Stir together peanut butter and butter in a mixing bowl until blended. Mix in chocolate and vanilla. Add flour mixture alternately with milk, beginning and ending with flour and mixing until smooth after each addition. Pour into prepared cake pans. Bake in 350° F. oven about 25 minutes or until cake tester inserted in center comes out clean.

Makes 16 servings

NOTE: To sour milk, add 1 tablespoon lemon juice or vinegar to 1 cup whole milk.

Variation: Peanut Butter Chocolate Cupcakes

Prepare batter according to Peanut Butter Chocolate Cake. Pour batter into 18 2½-by-1¼-inch cupcake pans lined with paper liners. Bake as directed for Peanut Butter Chocolate Cake.

Makes 18 cupcakes

Cream Cheese Pastry

EGG-FREE

This dough rolls out like a cook's dream come true—no drying up and cracking apart while handling.

1 3-ounce package cream cheese
½ cup butter
1 cup flour

Let cream cheese and butter come to room temperature. Combine them and add flour. Knead into a smooth dough. Chill for several hours. When ready to use, roll out two crusts. Place one crust in a pie pan, fill with desired filling, and top with the remaining crust. Crimp edges together to seal. If making a one-crust pie shell, place second crust in another pan and freeze until needed; or halve the recipe and prepare only one crust.

Makes 2 9-inch crusts

Apple Pie

EGG-FREE

Pies are a good dessert choice for those who suffer from egg allergies—they make up for some of the other goodies that must be missed!

2 prepared egg-free pie crusts (see index)
2 pounds tart apples, peeled and sliced
½ cup sugar
2 tablespoons flour
½ teaspoon cinnamon
¼ teaspoon nutmeg
⅛ teaspoon salt
1 tablespoon lemon juice
1 tablespoon butter

Place one pie crust into a 9-inch pie pan. Combine sliced apples, sugar, flour, cinnamon, nutmeg, and salt. Fill crust with mixture. Sprinkle with lemon juice and dot with butter. Top with second crust and crimp edges together. Prick with a fork to provide holes for steam to escape. Brush with milk. Bake at 425° F. for about 40 minutes, or until lightly browned.

Makes 8 servings

Cherry Pie

EGG-FREE

Substitute blueberries for the cherries and you'll have another recipe in your repertoire that will bring applause.

2 prepared 9-inch egg-free pie crusts (see index)
2 cups fresh sour cherries, pitted
2 tablespoons quick-cooking tapioca
1 tablespoon lemon juice
½ cup sugar
½ teaspoon cinnamon

Place first crust in a 9-inch pie pan. Combine cherries, tapioca, lemon juice, sugar, and cinnamon; mix gently but thoroughly. Let stand for 10 minutes. Fill pie shell and cover with second crust. Prick top crust with a fork to let steam escape. Brush top crust with milk, if desired. Bake in a 350° F. oven for 45 minutes, or until crust is lightly browned.

Makes 6–8 servings

Egg-Free Sugar Cookies

EGG-FREE

This is a simple dough cookie that makes a powdery mouthful for those times when a cookie is a must!

1½ cups sifted flour
¾ cup cornstarch
¾ cup confectioners' sugar
1 cup plus 2 tablespoons butter

Sift flour, cornstarch, and confectioners' sugar together in a large mixing bowl. Blend butter into dry ingredients, mixing until soft dough forms. Chill, if needed, until firm enough to handle. Shape into 1-inch balls. Place on ungreased cookie sheet, about 1½ inches apart. Flatten balls with lightly floured fork. Bake in 300° F. oven until edges of cookies are lightly browned, 20–25 minutes.

Makes about 4 dozen

Shortbread

EGG-FREE

This cookie bar is long on flavor for the egg-restricted palate. Dairy-free margarine or vegetable shortening may be used instead of butter.

2 cups sifted flour
1 cup cornstarch
Dash of salt
1 cup butter
½ cup sugar
Sugar

Sift flour, cornstarch, and salt together. Cream butter and ½ cup sugar until light and fluffy. Gradually add dry ingredients until dough is stiff enough to work with hands. Knead on lightly floured cloth or board until well blended and smooth. Press into 12-by-8-inch rectangle on baking sheet. Smooth over top. Score almost through with a knife into 1-by-2-inch rectangles; prick with a fork. Bake in a 325° F. oven for 30–40 minutes or until golden brown. Recut rectangles and sprinkle with sugar while still hot. Cool completely; remove from baking sheet. Store in an airtight container.

Makes 4 dozen rectangles

NOTE: For triangles, divide the 12-by-8-inch rectangle into 24 2-inch squares. Cut each square in half diagonally. Makes 4 dozen triangles.

6
The
Gluten-Free
Diet

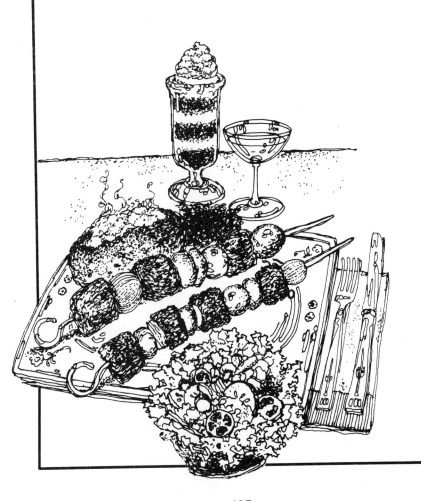

An allergy to wheat is probably the most difficult of all food sensitivities with which to cope. Wheat flour and its related gluten flours—rye, barley, and oatmeal—contain a factor that helps baked goods rise. When attempts are made to bake without any one of these grains, it is quite difficult to get the usual tender porous texture that is so moist and delicious.

Those who have Celiac-Sprue disease suffer from malabsorption in the lining of the small intestine due to an intolerance to gluten-gliaden in the gluten grains. Usually, these people must refrain from using any product that has gluten in it because the malabsorption leaves them with deficiencies in nutrients that are needed to provide good health. The most obvious symptoms in children are the effects on their ability to grow and thrive. Studies have shown that even when these children appear to have outgrown the disease by a cessation of symptoms, it is unwise to permit them to use gluten grains again. They are not actually cured, and the gluten may still be damaging the small intestine or may lead to gastrointestinal cancer and cancer of the esophagus. Today doctors put these individuals on a gluten-free diet for life, no matter how old they were when the sensitivity was discovered.

Some newly diagnosed celiac patients also show a lactose intolerance, particularly to milk, Many times, after these individuals have been on a gluten-free diet for several months, they are able to try hard cheese, buttermilk, yogurt, or cottage cheese. It's best to try these foods one at a time, waiting to see whether there is a reaction before proceeding to try the next one. Often, it is possible to reintroduce most dairy products into the diet of Celiac-Sprue patients, if done carefully.

The most accurate diagnosis of Celiac-Sprue is based on an intestinal biopsy that shows whether gluten is the culprit that causes damage to the small intestine. A second biopsy can be done after the individual has been on a strict gluten-free diet for two weeks, and it will usually reveal that the symptoms have disappeared. When such symptoms as stomach distress with gas and bloating, too frequent bowel movements, distended abdomen, exceptionally large bowel movements and/or diarrhea appear in children, a medical checkup to find the source of the problem is advised.

Adults may have symptoms of weight loss, anemia, edema, muscle cramps, profuse bleeding and hemorrhaging, bone pain and weakening of the bones, skin disorders, and gastrointestinal problems.

For those who are not afflicted with this disease but have been found to have a sensitivity to wheat and other glutens (rye, barley, and oats) that causes emotional mood swings or skin eruptions, it is important to have sublingual or intradermal tests performed by a qualified allergist to determine whether these substances in fact are contributing to the problems.

Whatever the cause of a sensitivity to gluten, it is necessary to avoid many manufactured food products that contain hidden gluten. Completely eliminate wheat flour, rye flour, barley, and oatmeal. Omit bran cereals, thick gravies (unless made with cornstarch), pancakes, waffles, breads, cookies, crackers, cakes, breaded foods, pasta, and even some hard candies. Don't order batter-fried foods outside the home because it is highly probable that wheat is in the batter or that the frying oil has been contaminated by other wheat-batter foods.

But don't despair. A gluten allergy may seem difficult to deal with at first, but other types of flour may be substituted for gluten flour with satisfactory results. Of course, most baked goods will not be as moist and spongy as gluten products, but there are ways to compensate.

Here are some tips to keep in mind:

- When adapting an egg-based baking recipe that calls for gluten, choose a suitable type of substitute flour, using the flour's flavor as your guide. Add an extra egg to recipes that contain less than 2 cups of wheat flour.
- When using rice flour, a smoother texture may be obtained by mixing the rice flour with the liquid called for in the recipe, bringing it to a boil, and then cooling it before adding it to the other ingredients.
- Soy flour cannot be used alone; it must be combined with another flour. Potato starch flour is a good combination.
- Coarse flours and meals (such as buckwheat or cornmeal) or a combination of several flours need not be sifted before measuring, but a combination of flours should be mixed thoroughly with other dry ingredients before adding to the batter or dough.
- Coarse meals and flours require more leavening than

wheat flour. Use 2½ teaspoons of baking powder for each cup of coarse flour.

- Nongluten breads tend to be crumbly. The use of buttermilk in place of milk will often result in a lighter, more finely textured product.
- Muffins and biscuits made of flours other than wheat often have a better (less crumbly) texture when made in small sizes and therefore are often more satisfactory than breads made with the same recipes.
- Cakes made with flours other than wheat have a tendency to be dry. Frosting and storing in a closed container will help preserve moisture.
- Cream of rice cereal in its uncooked state or crushed dry rice cereal makes an excellent breading for chicken, fish, cutlets, croquettes, and other coated patties.
- Note that when cornstarch is used as a *thickening* substitute for flour, you only need half the amount. This is also true for arrowroot, potato starch, and rice flour.

Substitutes for 1 Cup Wheat Flour

1 cup corn flour
¾ cup coarse cornmeal
¾ cup plus 3 tablespoons fine cornmeal
½ cup plus 2 tablespoons potato starch flour
¾ cup rice flour
1 cup soybean flour plus ¼ cup potato starch flour
1 cup millet flour
1 cup buckwheat flour

Substitutes for 1 Tablespoon Wheat Flour for Thickening

½ tablespoon cornstarch
½ tablespoon potato starch flour
½ tablespoon rice flour
½ tablespoon arrowroot starch
2 teaspoons quick cooking tapioca
1 tablespoon millet meal

As you browse through health food and foreign food stores you may find other types of flours that will suit your needs as well. Buckwheat flour is one that can be used if the label says that it is pure buckwheat (packages of buckwheat for pancakes and other baked goods contain some wheat flour to give them a gluten factor). Read the labels carefully to be sure that the contents are pure buckwheat and then use this flour when making pancakes, muffins or breads. You may also find such unique products as rice noodles in Oriental grocery stores, rhubarb flour in gourmet shops, and puffed rice crackers in ordinary, large grocery stores, which are suitable for open-faced sandwiches.

In this chapter you will find myriad gluten-free recipes that will show you how to bake with these alternate flours. Remember that the texture may not be the same as that given by a gluten flour, but each recipe will provide a satisfactory substitute. Once you have tried these recipes you may be inspired to experiment with some of your own favorites, using logical flour substitutes to see whether any of your own recipes can be converted and added to your list of baking possibilities for those sensitive to gluten. For additional gluten-free recipes, refer to Chapter 7 for multiple-allergy recipes.

APPETIZERS

Crab Puffs

GLUTEN-FREE
DAIRY-FREE

When you can't use a wheat cracker to prop up a mouthful of appetizer, use thick slices of cucumber instead. Crunchy and delicious!

1 egg white	**½ cup flaked cooked**
½ cup Mayonnaise	**crabmeat**
(see recipe)	**18 unpeeled ¼-inch-thick**
Paprika	**slices cucumber**

Beat egg white until stiff peaks form. Combine mayonnaise and flaked crabmeat; mix well. Fold mixture into egg whites. Pile mixture onto each slice of cucumber. Place on a cookie sheet and broil until lightly browned.

Makes 18 servings

Creamed Tuna-Cheese Spread

GLUTEN-FREE

If there is also an egg allergy, omit the mayonnaise and double up on the sour cream. This spread is good with vegetable crudités if rice crackers are also forbidden.

1 7-ounce can tuna, drained and flaked
1 3-ounce package cream cheese
2 tablespoons Mayonnaise (see recipe)
2 tablespoons dairy sour cream
1 tablespoon grated onion
½ teaspoon prepared white horseradish
¼ teaspoon Worcestershire sauce

Mix tuna and cream cheese. Add remaining ingredients and mix well. Chill. Place in a bowl for do-it-yourself spreading on rice crackers.

Makes 1½ cups

Chopped Chicken Livers

GLUTEN-FREE
DAIRY-FREE

This is the healthy way to cook livers for chopping. Don't fry them — simmer until tender and enjoy!

1 pound fresh chicken livers   **¼ teaspoon salt**
1 onion, sliced thin   **⅛ teaspoon pepper**
2 hard-cooked eggs

Place chicken livers and sliced onion in a large skillet; barely cover the bottom of the skillet with water. Cover and simmer for five minutes, turning the livers occasionally and adding more water if needed to keep the livers from sticking to the pan. Chop or grind livers, onions, and hard-cooked eggs together; stir in just enough pan juices to hold the mixture together. Add salt and pepper; chill until ready to use.

Makes about 1½ cups

Chopped Sardine Salad

GLUTEN-FREE

Those with a dairy restriction can omit the yogurt and double up on the mayonnaise.

2 3¾-ounce cans sardines, drained and broken into pieces
2 hard-cooked eggs, chopped
¼ cup chopped onion
2 tablespoons Mayonnaise (see recipe)
2 tablespoons plain yogurt
2 tablespoons white vinegar
1½ tablespoons sugar

Mix the sardines, egg, and onion together. Stir the mayonnaise, yogurt, vinegar, and sugar together; add this mixture to the sardine mixture and stir. Chill for several hours. Serve as an appetizer or sandwich filling.

Makes 1⅔ cups

Creamy Apple Dip

GLUTEN-FREE
EGG-FREE

Here's a novel dip to serve with crudités—a platter of crisp raw vegetables, such as broccoli buds, cauliflower flowerets, and carrot sticks. Delicious!

1 16-ounce can applesauce
1 cup sour cream
2 tablespoons minced onion
1 teaspoon Worcestershire sauce
½ teaspoon salt

Combine all ingredients and mix until well blended.

Makes 2½ cups

Creamy Olive Dip

GLUTEN-FREE
EGG-FREE

Use thick crisp potato chips or crisp French fried potatoes as the dipper for this zesty mixture, for the gluten-allergic. The combination is tantalizing!

1 cup sour cream
½ cup chopped green olives stuffed with pimiento
1 tablespoon white horseradish
1 3-ounce package cream cheese
½ teaspoon sugar
½ teaspoon salt
¼ teaspoon Worcestershire sauce

Stir sour cream, chopped olives, and horseradish together. Mash cream cheese and stir into the mixture until well blended. Add sugar, salt, and Worcestershire sauce.

Makes 2 cups

SOUPS

Avocado Yogurt Soup

GLUTEN-FREE
EGG-FREE

What a lovely way to serve an avocado, especially one that you have allowed to get a bit overripe! Serve very, very cold.

2 ripe avocados, peeled and seeded
2 teaspoons lemon juice
2 cups chicken broth
½ teaspoon onion salt
½ teaspoon celery salt
1 16-ounce carton plain yogurt
1 tablespoon chopped chives

Process avocados, lemon juice, chicken broth, onion salt, and celery salt in an electric blender or food processor. Add yogurt and process again. Chill thoroughly. Serve with a topping of chopped chives.

Makes 6 servings

Broccoli Bisque

GLUTEN-FREE
EGG-FREE

Here's a wonderful way to use up some extra cooked broccoli. Make it into a soup!

2 stalks fresh broccoli, trimmed (about ½ pound)
2 cups water
¼ teaspoon salt
¼ teaspoon dried dillweed
1 cup milk
1 teaspoon cornstarch

Place broccoli, water, salt, and dillweed in a saucepan. Cover and cook for 20 minutes, until broccoli is very soft. Pour entire contents of the saucepan into an electric blender or food processor and puree as fine as possible. Combine milk and cornstarch until free of lumps. Pour pureed broccoli back into the saucepan and stir in milk mixture. Cook over low heat, stirring constantly, until hot and slightly thickened.

Makes 4 servings

Spinach Soup

GLUTEN-FREE
EGG-FREE

Here's one that can be made dairy-free by substituting dairy-free margarine for the butter. Add extra nutmeg for those who savor it.

1 10-ounce package frozen chopped spinach
3 cups Chicken Broth (see recipe)
1 hot boiled medium potato, peeled
2 tablespoons butter
½ teaspoon salt
⅛ teaspoon pepper
⅛ teaspoon nutmeg

Cook spinach as directed on the package; drain. Put in blender or food processor with 1 cup of the chicken broth and the boiled potato. Blend until smooth. Pour remaining chicken broth into a saucepan; add butter, salt, pepper, and nutmeg. Stir in blended spinach mixture. Heat and serve.

Makes 6 servings

Potato Soup

GLUTEN-FREE
EGG-FREE

On a warm summer evening this tastes delicious served icy cold. Top with a sprinkling of fresh chopped chives.

4 large potatoes, peeled and
  diced
2 onions, diced
2 stalks celery, diced fine
1 sprig dillweed

2 cups water
1 teaspoon salt
3 cups milk
2 tablespoons butter

Place potatoes, onions, celery, dill, water, and salt in a saucepan; simmer for 20 minutes, or until potatoes are tender. Add milk and butter and stir until heated through.

Makes 4 servings

Fish Chowder

GLUTEN-FREE
EGG-FREE

Use just one kind of fish or a medley of several for a more interesting flavor.

2 tablespoons butter
1 large onion, sliced
1 pound fresh cod fillets (or other firm white fish),
    cut into chunks
3 cups water
1 bay leaf
2 large potatoes, peeled and diced
½ teaspoon salt
¼ teaspoon pepper
¼ teaspoon thyme
2 cups milk

Melt butter in a large saucepan; sauté onion until limp. Add fish, water, and bay leaf; simmer for 20 minutes, or until fish flakes easily. Transfer fish to a bowl. Add potatoes to the saucepan; add salt, pepper, and thyme. Cover and cook for 10 minutes, or until potatoes are soft. Return fish to the saucepan. Add milk. Heat but do not boil.

Makes 6 servings

ENTREES

Beef

Zesty Steak

GLUTEN-FREE
EGG-FREE

Omit the butter in favor of nondairy margarine for those who must. Enjoy the zesty flavor!

½ teaspoon dry mustard
½ teaspoon water
2 tablespoons Worcestershire sauce

2 tablespoons melted butter
1 sirloin steak (2–3 pounds)
½ teaspoon salt
⅛ teaspoon pepper

Mix mustard with water and let stand 10 minutes. Combine with Worcestershire sauce and melted butter. Broil steak on one side, turn and make several shallow slashes across top of steak. Pour butter mixture over steak and complete broiling. Season with salt and pepper and serve at once.

Makes 4–6 servings

Stuffed Cabbage

GLUTEN-FREE
DAIRY-FREE

This is a sweet and sour tangy dish. It tastes better the second day, so cook it ahead and refrigerate to give the flavors a chance to "marry."

1 large head of cabbage
1 pound lean ground beef
¼ cup uncooked white rice
1 small onion, grated
1 egg
2 tablespoons water

½ teaspoon salt
¼ teaspoon pepper
1 2-pound can tomatoes
Juice of 1 lemon
⅓ cup brown sugar
¼ teaspoon ginger

Parboil the cabbage just until you can remove the outer leaves easily. Discard the toughest outer leaves and trim the heavy center membrane of the remaining leaves to separate them. Combine the beef, rice, onion, egg, water, salt and pepper; mix well. Place a small amount of meat mixture at the trimmed membrane end of the cabbage leaf; roll forward once, fold the sides inward, and roll up to the top of the leaf. Repeat this until the meat mixture is used up. Cut up remaining cabbage and place in the bottom of a heavy saucepan or Dutch oven. Add tomatoes, the juice of the lemon, brown sugar, and ginger. Bring to a boil on top of the range, then cover and turn the heat low. Cook for about 2 hours, or until meat is tender.

Makes 6 servings

Stuffed Green Peppers

GLUTEN-FREE
DAIRY-FREE

Pick well-shaped large peppers for stuffing. This recipe freezes well after cooking, and reheats easily.

6 large green peppers	¼ teaspoon salt
1 pound lean ground beef	⅛ teaspoon pepper
1 egg	1 cup cooked rice
⅓ cup chopped onion plus	2 8-ounce cans tomato sauce
¼ cup chopped onion	½ teaspoon oregano

Cut off tops of peppers and remove the membranes and seeds. Boil in salted water for 2 minutes. Drain. Meanwhile, combine the beef, egg, ⅓ cup chopped onion, salt, pepper, and cooked rice; mix well. Stuff drained peppers with this mixture. Arrange stuffed peppers in a baking pan. Combine tomato sauce, ¼ cup chopped onion, and oregano; pour over and around the peppers. Bake in a 350° F. oven for 1 hour, basting occasionally with the sauce.

Makes 6 servings

Rice-Stuffed Flank Steak

GLUTEN-FREE
DAIRY-FREE

Here's a way to get a lot more mileage out of a small flank steak. Bake yourself a meal in one!

1½ cups cooked rice
1 egg, lightly beaten
2 tablespoons chopped parsley
1 teaspoon salt
1 flank steak (about 2 pounds)
¼ cup corn oil
4 cups beef stock or water
1 teaspoon dried oregano leaves
1 pound green beans, trimmed
1 pound mushrooms
3 tablespoons cornstarch
¼ cup water

Stir together rice, egg, and parsley. Sprinkle salt over steak. Spread rice mixture over steak to within 1 inch of edge. Roll up and tie securely with string. In a 5-quart Dutch oven, heat corn oil over medium heat. Add steak; brown well on all sides. Add beef stock and oregano. Cover; bring to a boil. Reduce heat; simmer 1 hour and 15 minutes. Add beans and mushrooms; continue cooking 20 minutes or until vegetables are crisp-tender. Transfer steak and vegetables to platter; keep warm. Stir together cornstarch and water until smooth. Stir into pan juices in Dutch oven. Bring to boil over medium heat, stirring constantly; boil 1 minute. Serve gravy with steak.

Makes 6–8 servings

Veal

Veal Balls Stroganoff

GLUTEN-FREE

The art of making a proper Stroganoff includes knowing how to keep the heat at a simmer so the creamy mixture will not curdle. In this version the veal balls are baked alone and then added to the sauce.

1 pound ground veal
2 tablespoons chopped parsley
1 teaspoon salt
2 eggs, beaten
½ cup coarsely shredded pared apple
1½ cups beef bouillon
⅛ teaspoon pepper
1 teaspoon dried dillweed
1 cup dairy sour cream
2 egg yolks, beaten
¼ cup finely chopped parsley
Hot cooked rice

Combine ground veal, parsley, salt, beaten eggs, and shredded apple. Shape into ¾-inch balls. Place on greased jelly roll pan and bake in a 350° F. oven for 20 minutes, or until cooked through. Meanwhile, heat bouillon, pepper, and dillweed together. Stir in sour cream, keeping heat low so it will not curdle. Spoon some of this mixture into the beaten egg yolks; return it gradually to the sour cream mixture. Heat until thick. Add veal balls. Sprinkle with chopped parsley and serve over hot cooked rice.

Makes 4 servings

Herbed Veal

GLUTEN-FREE

Be sure to roll the crispy rice cereal very fine so it will adhere to the egg batter. Makes a nice "breading."

4 thin slices veal cutlet, about 1½ pounds
½ cup crispy rice cold cereal, crushed fine
2 tablespoons butter
¼ teaspoon salt
⅛ teaspoon pepper
¼ cup nonfat dried milk
½ cup water
½ teaspoon dried thyme
½ teaspoon dried tarragon

Cover each piece of veal with waxed paper and pound with the flat side of a cleaver or wooden mallet until ⅛-inch thick. Dip each piece of veal into crushed rice cereal; coat well. Heat butter in a large skillet; add cutlets. Sprinkle with salt and pepper, and brown lightly on both sides. Remove cutlets to a warm platter. Stir dried milk into water; add thyme and tarragon and mix until smooth. Stir this mixture into the skillet; heat slowly over low heat, stirring in the brown crusty residue in the pan. Pour sauce over cutlets.

Makes 4 servings

Lamb

Lamb Shanks

GLUTEN-FREE
EGG-FREE

Exchange dairy-free margarine for the butter to create a sauce that may be served to the milk-sensitive among you. Don't omit the rosemary—it lifts the shanks out of the ordinary into the sublime!

4 lamb shanks
1 cup orange juice
2 tablespoons butter

1 tablespoon chopped parsley
½ teaspoon salt
½ teaspoon rosemary

Arrange lamb shanks in a small roasting pan. In a small saucepan, combine orange juice, butter, parsley, salt, and rosemary; heat and stir until butter melts. Brush half the mixture over the lamb shanks. Roast 1 hour in a 350° F. oven, basting occasionally with remaining sauce. Continue roasting until fork-tender.

Makes 4 servings

Lamb Kebobs

GLUTEN-FREE
EGG-FREE

If you must omit the yogurt, use 1 cup of red wine in its place. Use dairy-free margarine in place of the butter. A different taste, but good nevertheless!

1 cup plain yogurt
1 tablespoon lemon juice
2 tablespoons grated onion
1 teaspoon minced dillweed
½ teaspoon salt
2 pounds lamb, cubed
8 small onions, boiled
8 mushroom caps
2 tablespoons melted butter

Combine yogurt, lemon juice, onion, dillweed, and salt. Stir in lamb cubes; marinate in refrigerator for several hours. Alternate lamb cubes, onions, and mushroom caps on skewers. Place in a flat pan. Brush with melted butter. Broil 6 minutes. Turn and brush with remaining melted butter; broil 6 minutes more, or until tender.

Makes 4 servings

Poultry

Broiled Chicken Rosemary

GLUTEN-FREE
EGG-FREE

Here's an easy and fast way to broil delectable chicken. Use dairy-free margarine if necessary.

2 small broiler chickens	¼ teaspoon salt
(about 2 pounds each), split	⅛ teaspoon pepper
2 tablespoons melted butter	¼ teaspoon rosemary
2 tablespoons lemon juice	

Place halves of chicken on a broiling pan, skin side down. Combine butter, lemon juice, salt, pepper, and rosemary, stirring well. Brush half of this mixture on top of chicken and broil for 10 minutes. Turn chicken, brush the skin side with the remaining mixture, and broil for 10 minutes more, or until tender.

Makes 4 servings

Orange-Roasted Chicken

GLUTEN-FREE
EGG-FREE

Orange and chicken are so compatible! Brush with dairy-free margarine instead of butter if there is a milk allergy at your house.

1 roasting chicken (about	2 small oranges, halved
5 pounds)	¼ cup cornstarch
4 tablespoons butter, melted	2 cups orange juice
1 teaspoon salt	1 cup Chicken Broth
¼ teaspoon pepper	(see recipe)
½ teaspoon dried rosemary	1 tablespoon brown sugar
leaves	

Place chicken in a roasting pan. Brush with butter. Season with salt, pepper, and rosemary. Place oranges in the cavity of the chicken. Tie the legs together. Bake in a 325° F. oven, basting occasionally, about 2½ hours, or until skin is browned and leg joint moves easily. Remove chicken to platter. Measure fat drippings and return ¼ cup to roasting pan. Sprinkle cornstarch into pan drippings. Stir and cook over medium heat just until smooth; remove from heat. Gradually stir in orange juice, chicken stock, and sugar until smooth. Bring to a boil over medium heat, stirring constantly, and boil 2 minutes. Serve gravy over chicken.

Makes about 6 servings

Chicken Stroganoff

GLUTEN-FREE

Be sure to follow the directions for stirring so that this will turn out smooth and tasty.

3 whole chicken breasts, boned and halved	1 teaspoon salt
¼ cup cornstarch	⅛ teaspoon pepper
1 tablespoon butter	½ teaspoon dried dillweed
2 tablespoons salad oil	1 cup dairy sour cream
¼ cup finely chopped onion	2 egg yolks, beaten
1½ cups chicken broth	¼ cup finely chopped parsley
	3 cups hot cooked rice

Dust chicken lightly with cornstarch. Heat butter and oil in a skillet; add onions and chicken (skin side down) and cook until golden brown, turning chicken once. Add broth, salt, pepper, and dillweed. Cover and simmer 15 minutes, or until chicken is tender. Transfer chicken to a warm platter. Stir sour cream into the broth. Remove some of the sour cream mixture and stir into the beaten egg yolks; gradually stir this mixture back into the sour cream mixture in the skillet. Simmer until thickened, but do not allow to boil. Pour over chicken. Sprinkle with chopped parsley. Serve over hot rice.

Makes 6 servings

Middle Eastern Chicken

GLUTEN-FREE
EGG-FREE

Butter can be replaced by dairy-free margarine in this eggplant-chicken duet. Funny how eggplant always takes on the flavor of whatever it is paired with!

2 broiler chickens, cut into serving pieces
1 teaspoon salt
¼ teaspoon paprika
2 tablespoons butter
2 tablespoons salad oil
2 onions, chopped
2 cloves garlic, minced
2 8-ounce cans tomato sauce
1 teaspoon dried thyme
1 teaspoon dried basil
½ teaspoon Tabasco sauce
2 medium eggplants, peeled and diced

Sprinkle chicken pieces with salt and paprika. Melt butter in a large skillet; add oil, onion, and garlic. Cook until onion is translucent. Brown chicken pieces. Combine tomato sauce, thyme, basil, and Tabasco; add to skillet. Simmer, covered, for 15 minutes. Add eggplant and cook, covered, 10 minutes longer, or until chicken is tender.

Makes 8 servings

Honey-Broiled Chicken

GLUTEN-FREE
EGG-FREE

You may replace the butter with dairy-free margarine. Wait until you taste this bit of honey-sweetened chicken!

2 broiler chickens (about
   3 pounds each), split
Juice of 2 lemons
½ teaspoon salt
¼ teaspoon pepper

¼ cup honey
4 tablespoons butter
1 teaspoon dried tarragon
1 clove garlic, peeled
   and mashed

Sprinkle both sides of broiler halves with lemon juice, salt, and pepper. Brush both sides lightly with honey. Blend butter, tarragon, and garlic together. Spread half of the mixture over the side of chicken facing the broiler; broil 10 minutes. Turn and spread the remaining mixture on the other side of the chicken. Broil an additional 10 minutes, or until done.

Makes 4 servings

Fried Chicken

GLUTEN-FREE
DAIRY-FREE

Omit the eggs if you must, but don't expect to have a thick crust. Add a bit of sweet paprika to the cornstarch if you want a perkier flavor.

1 fryer chicken, cut up
½ teaspoon salt
⅛ teaspoon pepper
2 eggs
1 tablespoon water
¾ cup cornstarch
1 cup corn oil

Sprinkle chicken with salt and pepper. Beat eggs and water together. Dip chicken into egg mixture, then into cornstarch to coat evenly. Dip into egg mixture again; drain off excess. Pour corn oil into a large deep skillet. Heat over medium heat. Carefully put chicken into hot oil to avoid spattering. Cook, turning once, 25–35 minutes, or until light golden brown and tender. Drain on absorbent paper.

Makes 4 servings

Chicken Almond Salad

GLUTEN-FREE
DAIRY-FREE

Almonds and celery give crunch to this chicken salad. Add a dash of tarragon, if desired.

1½ cups finely chopped cooked chicken
3 tablespoons slivered blanched almonds
¼ cup diced celery
2 tablespoons grated carrot
½ cup Mayonnaise (see recipe)
¼ teaspoon salt
Dash of pepper

Combine chicken, almonds, carrot, mayonnaise, salt, and pepper. Use as a salad or as a sandwich spread.

Makes 2½ cups

Creamy Chicken and Mushrooms

GLUTEN-FREE
EGG-FREE

This becomes Chicken à la King if you add some peas and pimiento. Delicious when served over cooked rice.

6 tablespoons butter
8 ounces mushrooms, sliced
3 tablespoons cornstarch
1 teaspoon salt
¼ teaspoon pepper
½ teaspoon onion salt
3 cups milk
2 cups cooked diced chicken or turkey

In a medium saucepan, melt 2 tablespoons of the butter. Add mushrooms and cook over medium heat about 3 minutes, or until tender. Remove mushrooms, reserving pan juices. Heat remaining butter with juices in saucepan. Remove from heat. Add cornstarch, salt, pepper, and onion salt, stirring until smooth. Gradually add milk. Cook over medium heat, stirring constantly, until mixture comes to a boil. Boil 1 minute. Stir in chicken and mushrooms until well mixed.

Makes 6 servings

Rock Cornish Hens

GLUTEN-FREE
EGG-FREE

There's always something special about Rock Cornish hens. The lemon ensures a fresh flavor. Use dairy-free margarine instead of butter, if dairy products are a problem.

3 Rock Cornish Hens (1½ pounds each)
1 lemon, halved
¾ teaspoon salt
¼ teaspoon pepper
3 tablespoons melted butter
Paprika

Rinse and dry hens. (Each hen should serve 2. If hens are under 1 pound each, prepare one for each person.) Rub inside and out with lemon halves. Cut up lemon and tuck pieces into the cavities of the hens. Season hens with salt and pepper. Brush with melted butter and dust lightly with paprika. Roast in a 350° F. oven for 45 minutes to 1 hour, depending on size. Serve at once.

Makes 6 servings

Roast Turkey with Orange Glaze

GLUTEN-FREE
EGG-FREE

If you squeeze the orange juice yourself, be sure to tuck the leftover rinds into the turkey cavity—they will give extra flavor at no extra cost. Use dairy-free margarine instead of butter for those sensitive to milk.

1 large roasting turkey (thawed, if frozen)
1 teaspoon salt
1 teaspoon paprika
¼ cup butter
½ cup orange juice

Clean turkey and season with salt and paprika. Melt butter in a small saucepan; stir in orange juice. Use about a fourth of this mixture to brush all over the skin of the turkey. Place turkey on a rack in a large roasting pan. Roast in a 325° F. oven for approximately 20 minutes to the pound, uncovered for the first hour and then loosely tented with aluminum foil for the remaining cooking time. Baste turkey every half hour with the remaining butter sauce. To test for doneness, jiggle the drumstick. It will move easily when the bird is thoroughly cooked. (Or use a meat thermometer inserted deep into the thickest part of the white meat, near the thigh. When it reaches a temperature of 190° F. the bird is done.) To make gravy, remove the bird from the pan and pour in a small amount of boiling water, scraping up the drippings that have stuck to the pan. Set pan over medium heat and bring to a simmer, stirring until you have as much gravy as you require. The turkey will benefit from resting while you are preparing the gravy—it will be easier to carve about 20 minutes after being removed from the oven.

Fish

Sole Granada

GLUTEN-FREE

Does this sound like an implausible combination? When you taste this banana and fish combo you'll have to agree that it's a delight.

4 fillets of sole (about 2 pounds)
¼ cup lemon juice
¼ cup water
1 tablespoon thinly sliced scallions
½ teaspoon salt
⅛ teaspoon pepper
1 cup Blender Hollandaise Sauce (see recipe)
2 medium bananas

Place sole fillets in a large skillet. Add lemon juice, water, scallions, salt, and pepper. Simmer for 3 minutes, frequently spooning liquid over fish. Transfer fillets to an ovenproof serving platter. Peel bananas and cut in half lengthwise; place one banana half on each fish fillet. Cover with Hollandaise Sauce. Place under a broiler for 2–3 minutes, or until sauce is golden.

Makes 4 servings

Sole Rolls

GLUTEN-FREE
EGG-FREE

For a change of pace, mash a whole pimiento into the cream cheese filling. Pink and pretty!

4 fillets of sole (about 2 pounds)
1 3-ounce package chive cream cheese
2 tablespoons milk
½ teaspoon salt
⅛ teaspoon pepper
⅛ teaspoon paprika
¼ cup light cream

Spread one side of sole slices with chive cream cheese softened with milk. Roll up. Place in buttered baking dish. Sprinkle with salt, pepper, and paprika. Pour cream around fish. Bake in a 375° F. oven for 20 minutes.

Makes 4 servings

Flounder Parmigiana

GLUTEN-FREE
EGG-FREE

For extra flavor, sprinkle the fish with lemon juice about two hours before cooking. Refrigerate and let the lemon tenderize the fish tissue!

1 pound fillets of flounder
2 tablespoons lemon juice
½ teaspoon salt
⅛ teaspoon pepper
1 tablespoon grated onion
½ teaspoon oregano
2 tablespoons grated Parmesan cheese
1 tablespoon butter

Arrange flounder fillets on a broiling pan. Sprinkle with lemon juice. Season with salt and pepper. Add grated onion, oregano, and then grated cheese. Dot with butter. Broil for 10–15 minutes, or until fish flakes easily.

Makes 4 servings

Mushroom-Sauced Flounder

GLUTEN-FREE
EGG-FREE

This can easily be made milk-free by substituting dairy-free margarine for butter. A simple fish dish that satisfies.

4 slices fillet of flounder
½ cup lemon juice
¼ teaspoon salt
⅛ teaspoon pepper
3 tablespoons butter
¼ pound fresh mushrooms, sliced
¼ teaspoon dried dillweed

Arrange fillets of flounder in one layer in a flat baking dish. Pour lemon juice over and refrigerate, covered, for at least 1 hour. When ready to broil, sprinkle with the salt and pepper; slip under the broiler for about 10 minutes, or until fish flakes easily. Meanwhile, melt butter in a skillet and sauté mushrooms for several minutes until golden and limp. Add dillweed. Spoon over broiled fish and serve at once.

Makes 4 servings

Broiled Halibut

GLUTEN-FREE
EGG-FREE

Omit the sour cream for those with a milk allergy.

1½ pounds halibut fillets
2 tablespoons lemon juice
¼ teaspoon salt
¼ teaspoon dillweed
½ cup dairy sour cream
½ teaspoon paprika

Arrange halibut fillets in a single layer in a broiling pan. Sprinkle with lemon juice, salt, and dillweed. Spread a thin coating of sour cream over the top of each piece of fish. Sprinkle with paprika. Broil for about 15 minutes. The fish is cooked through if it flakes easily when touched with a fork.

Makes 4 servings

Spanish Mackerel with Pineapple Sauce

GLUTEN-FREE
EGG-FREE

If you've never cooked Spanish mackerel, here's a good recipe for your first try. Dairy-sensitive people can replace butter with dairy-free margarine.

4 Spanish mackerel fillets
½ teaspoon salt
⅛ teaspoon pepper
2 tablespoons melted butter
1 tablespoon cornstarch
1 cup pineapple juice

Arrange fish in a flat baking dish. Season with salt and

pepper. Brush with 1 tablespoon of the melted butter. Broil for 6–8 minutes, or until the fish flakes easily. Meanwhile, stir the remaining tablespoon of melted butter with cornstarch in a saucepan over low heat; cook until thick and bubbling. Remove from heat and gradually stir in the pineapple juice. Cook and stir constantly until the mixture is thick and smooth. Pour over the cooked fish and serve at once.

Makes 4 servings

Salmon Mousse

GLUTEN-FREE

Many salmon mousse recipes are propped up with gelatin and served cold, but this one makes it without gelatin and is a fluffy delight for a hot dinner.

1 pound canned salmon
½ teaspoon salt
⅛ teaspoon pepper
½ teaspoon dried dillweed
2 teaspoons lemon juice
½ cup heavy cream, whipped
3 egg whites, beaten stiff

Drain salmon and remove skin and bones. Mash with salt, pepper, dillweed, and lemon juice. Fold in whipped cream. Fold in stiffly beaten egg whites. Spoon the mixture into a buttered 1-quart ring mold. Place the ring mold in a pan of water in a 350° F. oven. Bake for 20–25 minutes, or until firm to the touch. Turn out of the mold and serve hot.

Makes 4–6 servings

Broiled Scallops

GLUTEN-FREE
EGG-FREE

Here's an easy way to prepare scallops—takes just a few moments from broiler to table. Substitute dairy-free margarine for butter, if desired.

4 tablespoons butter	⅛ teaspoon pepper
1½ pounds fresh scallops	1 tablespoon minced parsley
2 tablespoons minced scallions	¼ cup lemon juice
½ teaspoon salt	

Place butter in a flat baking dish. Heat in the oven until the butter melts. Add the scallops in a single layer. Scatter the minced scallions around the scallops. Add salt, pepper, and parsley. Broil for 5 minutes, or until tender. Just before removing from the oven, sprinkle the scallops with the lemon juice and return for 1 more minute.

Makes 4 servings

Shrimp Fried Rice

GLUTEN-FREE
DAIRY-FREE

No need to go to a Chinese restaurant for this Oriental specialty. Those on an egg-free regimen can omit the eggs and still have an interesting shrimp/rice dish.

1 pound shrimp (fresh or frozen and thawed), deveined and
    diced
2 tablespoons chopped scallions
1 teaspoon cornstarch
1 teaspoon salt
¼ teaspoon pepper
¼ cup corn oil
3 cups cooked rice
2 eggs, slightly beaten
1½ teaspoons salt

In a large bowl, stir together shrimp, scallions, cornstarch, 1 teaspoon salt, and the pepper. In a wok or skillet, heat corn oil over medium-high heat. Add shrimp mixture. Cook, stirring constantly, 3–5 minutes, or until shrimp turns pink. Remove from wok with a slotted spoon. In a medium bowl, stir together cooked rice, eggs, and remaining salt. Place in the wok. Stir and cook over medium-high heat, about 2 minutes, until egg is cooked. Add shrimp mixture and cook, stirring constantly, until heated.

Makes 6 servings

Tuna Lentil Creole

GLUTEN-FREE
EGG-FREE

This casserole can be converted for the milk-sensitive by using dairy-free margarine in place of butter. Lentils are an excellent source of extra protein when combined with rice!

1 cup dried lentils
2½ teaspoons salt
3 tablespoons butter
2 cups chopped green pepper
¾ cup chopped onion
1 28-ounce can tomatoes

1 10-ounce package frozen
  sliced okra, thawed
1 teaspoon brown sugar
⅛ teaspoon Tabasco sauce
2 7-ounce cans tuna, drained
Hot cooked rice

In a medium saucepan, cover lentils with water; add 2 teaspoons of the salt and bring to a boil. Cook uncovered over medium heat for 1½ hours, adding additional water if necesary, until lentils are tender. Drain and set lentils aside. Melt butter in a large saucepan; add green pepper, onion, and okra and cook 2–3 minutes over medium heat. Add tomatoes, sugar, Tabasco, the remaining ½ teaspoon salt, and the drained lentils. Cover and simmer 30 minutes. Add tuna and simmer 10 minutes. Serve over hot rice.

Makes 6 servings

Tuna and Brown Rice

GLUTEN-FREE
EGG-FREE

Ripe black olives and pecans are the ingredients that give flair to this canned tuna casserole.

1¼ cups uncooked brown rice
3 cups water
¼ cup butter
1 cup chopped celery
½ cup chopped pecans
½ cup chopped ripe olives
3 tablespoons chopped chives
1 teaspoon salt

1½ teaspoons dried tarragon
½ cup shredded sharp
  cheddar cheese
½ cup plain yogurt
1 cup milk
2 7-ounce cans tuna,
  drained

Place brown rice and water in a large saucepan. Bring to a boil, reduce heat, cover, and cook until rice is tender and water is absorbed, about 45 minutes. Remove from heat and add butter, celery, pecans, olives, chives, salt, tarragon, shredded cheese, yogurt, and milk; mix well. Stir in tuna. Turn into a buttered 2-quart casserole and bake in a 300° F. oven for 45 minutes.

Makes 6 servings

Seafood Herb Dressing

GLUTEN-FREE

Those afflicted with a milk allergy but not an egg sensitivity can use 1 cup of mayonnaise and omit the yogurt. Great with all kinds of fish!

½ cup Mayonnaise (see recipe)
½ cup yogurt
1 tablespoon finely chopped
  parsley

1½ teaspoons chopped chives
1½ teaspoons dried tarragon
  leaves
½ teaspoon chopped dillweed

Mix together the mayonnaise and yogurt. Add the parsley,

chives, tarragon, and dillweed. Chill at least 2 hours before serving.

Makes 1 cup

EGG DISHES

Banana Egg Nog

GLUTEN-FREE

If you can't have most cereals and breads because of a gluten allergy, here's a fast and nourishing breakfast drink to make in the electric blender.

2 cups milk	**2 eggs**
3 ripe bananas	**1 tablespoon honey**

Combine all ingredients in an electric blender (or food processor) container. Cover and process at high speed for 1 minute. Serve at once.

Makes 3 servings

Deviled Eggs

GLUTEN-FREE

If you replace the sour cream with mayonnaise, you can serve this to the dairy-sensitive diner. The pinch of mustard gives it a zippy flavor!

6 peeled hard-cooked eggs	**⅛ teaspoon dry mustard**
1 tablespoon dairy sour cream	**⅛ teaspoon pepper**
¼ teaspoon salt	**⅛ teaspoon paprika**

Cut eggs in half lengthwise. Scoop out the yolks and place in a bowl, reserving the whites. Mash the yolks; add sour cream, salt, dry mustard, and pepper, mixing well. Spoon mixture back into the reserved whites, mounding the yolks carefully in their cavities. Sprinkle paprika over the yolks. Chill until ready to serve.

Makes 12

Eggs Florentine

GLUTEN-FREE

This is a lovely dish to make for a brunch or luncheon because it can be prepared ahead of time. Just heat and eat!

2 tablespoons butter
¼ cup chopped onion
1 10-ounce package frozen chopped spinach, cooked and
    drained
1 tablespoon cornstarch
½ cup milk
4 hard-cooked eggs, halved lengthwise
1 recipe White Sauce (below)
½ cup fine dry gluten-free breadcrumbs (see recipe)
2 tablespoons grated Parmesan cheese
2 tablespoons melted butter

Melt 2 tablespoons butter in a 1½-quart saucepan over medium heat. Add onion; sauté, stirring frequently, until tender. Add spinach. Mix cornstarch and milk. Stir into spinach. Bring to a boil, stirring constantly, and boil 1 minute. Turn into a 10-by-6-by-1¾-inch baking dish. Place egg halves on top. Cover with White Sauce. Toss breadcrumbs and cheese with melted butter. Sprinkle over egg mixture. Bake in a 350° F. oven about 20 minutes, or until casserole is heated through and breadcrumbs are browned.

Makes 4 servings

White Sauce

4 tablespoons butter   ¼ teaspoon pepper
2 tablespoons cornstarch   2 cups milk
1 teaspoon salt

Melt butter in a small saucepan. Mix in cornstarch, salt, and pepper. Remove from heat. Gradually add milk, stirring until smooth. Cook over medium heat, stirring constantly, until mixture comes to boil. Boil 1 minute.

Makes 2 cups

Egg and Cheese Florentine

GLUTEN-FREE

This elegant dish is deceptively simple to make.

1 10-ounce package frozen spinach	4 eggs
1 cup creamy cottage cheese	½ teaspoon salt

Cook spinach according to directions on the package; drain well. Combine spinach with cottage cheese. Spoon into 4 greased individual baking dishes. In the center of each, make a depression large enough to hold one raw egg. Break an egg into each center. Bake in a 350° F. oven for 15 minutes, or until egg is firm to your taste. Sprinkle with salt and serve.

Makes 4 servings

Omelets

Cheese and Chive Omelet

GLUTEN-FREE

If you miss the crunch of toast with eggs, serve this omelet with rice cake discs—available at most supermarkets or health food stores.

3 eggs	3 tablespoons coarsely chopped white cheddar cheese
1 tablespoon cold water	1 tablespoon chopped chives
¼ teaspoon salt	
1 tablespoon butter	

Beat eggs, water, and salt together. Melt butter in a small skillet; pour egg mixture into skillet. As egg solidifies, gently push the edges toward the middle, allowing the liquid egg to run to the edges. While still wet, sprinkle with cheese and chopped chives. Cover for a moment. Roll omelet out of the pan onto a platter.

Makes 2 servings

Strawberry Cheese Omelet

GLUTEN-FREE

Here's a perfect Sunday night quickie supper. You'll think you're eating dessert!

1 1-pound package frozen strawberries, thawed
2 3-ounce packages cream cheese, softened
8 eggs
½ cup water
1 teaspoon salt
4 teaspoons butter

Drain strawberries, reserving liquid. Blend cream cheese with ¼ cup strawberry liquid. Set aside. For each omelet, beat 2 eggs with 2 tablespoons water and ¼ teaspoon salt. Heat 1 teaspoon butter in a small skillet; pour in egg mixture. With a spatula, carefully draw cooked portions at edges toward center so that uncooked portions flow to the bottom. When eggs are set and surface is still moist, remove from heat and spread ¼ of the cheese mixture over half of the omelet. Fold and slip out onto serving plate. Place ¼ of the strawberries on top of omelet and serve. Repeat until you have made 4 omelets.

Makes 4 servings

Onion-Pepper Omelet

GLUTEN-FREE

Use dairy-free margarine for the milk-sensitive. Add some chopped tomato to the skillet for variety. The filling cooks into the eggs.

3 tablespoons butter
1 onion, sliced thin
1 green pepper, seeded and diced
4 eggs
1 tablespoon cold water
¼ teaspoon salt

Melt butter in a skillet. Add onions and green pepper; sauté until limp. Beat eggs well; add water and salt. Pour eggs over onions and pepper and cook until solidified. With a spatula, roll omelet out of the pan onto a warm platter.

Makes 2 servings

Vegetable Omelet

GLUTEN-FREE
DAIRY-FREE

Don't be limited by the vegetables listed here. If you want to add some thinly sliced celery, leftover cooked green beans, or even broccoli flowerets–do it!

2 tablespoons margarine
1 onion, sliced thin
2 sweet green peppers, seeded and sliced thin
2 small tomatoes, cut into small chunks
4 eggs
¼ teaspoon salt
1 tablespoon cold water

Melt margarine in a skillet. Sauté onion and green pepper until limp. Add tomatoes and cook over low heat, stirring occasionally, until limp. Beat eggs, salt, and water together; pour over cooked vegetables. Gently push solidified egg toward the center to let liquid egg flow to the edges. Cover for a moment. Using a spatula, lift up the omelet on one side of the pan and roll it out onto a platter. Cut in half and serve.

Makes 2 servings

Cottage Cheese Puffs

GLUTEN-FREE

Plan to serve this as soon as it is ready. As with all souffle-type dishes, what puffs up quickly sinks down!

3 eggs, separated
1 cup creamed cottage cheese
1 teaspoon grated onion
½ cup orange juice
½ teaspoon salt
½ teaspoon dry mustard
⅛ teaspoon pepper
½ teaspoon grated orange rind
¼ teaspoon cream of tartar

Combine egg yolks, cottage cheese, onion, orange juice, salt, dry mustard, pepper, and orange rind; beat well. In another bowl, beat egg whites with cream of tartar until stiff but not dry. Fold yolk mixture into egg whites. Spoon into 4 10-ounce individual soufflé dishes. Bake in a preheated 350° F. oven 20–30 minutes, or until top is puffed and slightly browned and the tip of a knife inserted in the center comes out clean.

Makes 4 servings

Egg Puffs

GLUTEN-FREE

Be sure that the egg whites are beaten until peaks stand up very stiff. That's the secret to preventing a puff that flops!

2 tablespoons butter
3 tablespoons cornstarch
½ teaspoon salt
⅛ teaspoon pepper
1 cup milk
4 eggs, separated

Melt butter in a saucepan. Remove from heat; stir in cornstarch, salt, and pepper. Gradually stir in milk until smooth. Bring to a boil, over medium heat, stirring constantly, and boil 1 minute. Remove from heat and pour over egg yolks, mixing well. Beat egg whites until stiff; fold into egg yolk mixture. Pour into an ungreased 8-inch square pan. Place the pan in a larger pan of warm water and bake in a 350° F. oven 45–50 minutes, or until knife inserted in the center comes out clean. Cut into squares and serve at once.

Makes 4–6 servings

Pancakes and Crêpes

Wheat-Free Crêpes

GLUTEN-FREE

These crêpes can be filled with fruit, seafood, or chicken. Freeze extras between sheets of wax paper.

2 eggs
¾ cup milk
6 tablespoons cornstarch
1 tablespoon corn oil
¾ teaspoon baking powder
½ teaspoon salt

Beat eggs; add milk, cornstarch, oil, baking powder, and salt. Mix until smooth. Lightly butter a 6-inch skillet and place over low heat. Spoon 2–3 tablespoons of batter into skillet and quickly tilt the pan so the bottom is covered with batter. When crêpe is a solid circle and is browned lightly on the bottom, tap it out upside down onto a clean dish towel if it is to be filled and baked in a sauce. If not, turn crêpe and brown the other side before tapping out onto towel. Butter skillet again and repeat until all batter is used.

Makes about 12

Pineapple-Fritters

GLUTEN-FREE

Rice flour alone would have a gritty texture, but when combined with potato flour it makes a pretty fine fritter.

½ cup potato flour
½ cup rice flour
1½ teaspoons baking powder
2 tablespoons light brown sugar
¼ teaspoon salt
½ cup milk
1 egg, lightly beaten
¼ cup canned water-packed crushed pineapple, well drained

Combine potato flour, rice flour, baking powder, sugar, and salt. Stir in milk, egg, and pineapple. Drop by tablespoonfuls onto a hot greased griddle and cook until browned on both sides. Or drop into hot fat and cook until browned.

Makes 4–6 servings

Cornmeal Rice Pancakes

GLUTEN-FREE

People with a gluten allergy think they'll never be able to have pancakes again. Here's proof that it can be done deliciously!

1 cup uncooked rice
2½ cups milk
⅓ cup cornmeal
3 eggs, beaten
½ teaspoon salt
1 teaspoon freshly grated lemon rind

Place rice and milk in the top of a double boiler, over hot water, and cook until rice is soft and has absorbed most of the milk. Stir in cornmeal. Cool for 10 minutes. Stir in beaten eggs, salt, and lemon rind; mix well. Drop by tablespoonfuls onto a hot greased griddle or skillet; brown on one side, turn and brown the other side.

Makes 4 servings

Blueberry Rice Pancakes

GLUTEN-FREE

The baking powder gives a glutenlike quality to this pancake. The berries make it all worthwhile!

2 eggs
1 cup milk
¾ cup rice flour
1½ teaspoons baking powder
1 tablespoon light brown sugar
½ cup fresh blueberries, washed and dried

Beat eggs and half of the milk together. Add flour, baking powder, and sugar. Add remaining milk. (If batter is too stiff, add a few more tablespoons of milk.) Add blueberries. Spoon batter into 4-inch rounds on a hot greased griddle. Cook on one side until lightly browned, then flip to brown on the other side.

Makes 4 servings

VEGETABLES

Asparagus with Pecan Butter Sauce

GLUTEN-FREE
EGG-FREE

This asparagus becomes dairy-free when butter is replaced by dairy-free margarine. A good trick when cooking asparagus is to stand the bunch (thick stems down) in the bottom of a double boiler. Then invert the top pan over the asparagus tips and create a tall pot.

1 pound fresh asparagus, trimmed
2 tablespoons butter
⅓ cup coarsely chopped pecans
1 tablespoon lemon juice

Plunge fresh asparagus into boiling water for 1 minute. Then plunge asparagus into a waiting bowl of ice water until ready to cook. (This method preserves the bright green color for several hours.) Cook asparagus covered with water, or place it in a steaming unit, for 10–15 minutes, or until fork-tender. Drain. Melt butter in a skillet; add chopped pecans and sauté for a minute. Stir in lemon juice. Pour sauce over asparagus and serve at once.

Makes 4–6 servings

Broccoli with Sesame Sauce

GLUTEN-FREE
EGG-FREE

It's the little touches of seeds and herbs that turn an ordinary vegetable into something special. Exchange dairy-free margarine for butter, if needed.

4 stalks fresh broccoli
  (about 1 pound)
Water

½ teaspoon salt
2 tablespoons sesame seeds
3 tablespoons butter

Trim broccoli and cut lengthwise into serving pieces. Place in a saucepan with 2 inches of water; add salt. Cover and cook for 8–10 minutes, or until tender. Drain and place on a serving platter. Brown sesame seeds lightly in a skillet, then add butter and toss with seeds as it melts. Pour over broccoli.

Makes 4 servings

Brussels Sprouts Marjoram

GLUTEN-FREE
EGG-FREE

If you can purchase fresh Brussels sprouts, do so! Use dairy-free margarine for butter if you are cooking for a milk-sensitive person.

**1 10-ounce package frozen Brussels sprouts or 1 pint fresh
    Brussels sprouts
1 cup water
1 teaspoon chopped parsley
½ teaspoon salt
¼ teaspoon dried marjoram
⅛ teaspoon white pepper
1 tablespoon butter**

Cut large Brussels sprouts in half lengthwise and place in a saucepan with the water, parsley, salt, marjoram, and pepper. Cook for 5 minutes or until tender but not mushy. Drain. Toss lightly with butter and serve.

Makes 4 servings

Eggplant-Tomato Bake

GLUTEN-FREE
EGG-FREE

The milk-sensitive can enjoy this recipe by omitting the cheese and using dairy-free margarine in place of butter. If desired, crush crispy rice cereal and sprinkle on top.

1 eggplant (about 1 pound)	½ teaspoon dried basil
3 large tomatoes	2 tablespoons grated
½ cup tomato juice	Parmesan cheese
½ teaspoon salt	2 tablespoons butter

Peel and slice eggplant lengthwise into ¼-inch slices. Peel and slice the tomatoes. Pour half the tomato juice over the bottom of a baking dish. Arrange half the eggplant slices side by side in the baking dish. Cover with tomato slices. Season with salt and basil. Layer another tier of eggplant slices and top with remaining tomato slices. Season with salt and basil. Sprinkle with grated Parmesan cheese and dot with butter. Pour remaining tomato juice around the sides. Bake in a 350° F. oven for 1 hour, or until eggplant is fork-tender.

Makes 6 servings

Carrots in Parsley Sauce

GLUTEN-FREE
EGG-FREE

A food processor will slice these carrots in jig time! Good equipment helps good cooking. Use dairy-free margarine in place of butter, if desired.

2½ cups sliced pared carrots	2 tablespoons chopped
½ cup water	fresh parsley
2 tablespoons butter	¼ teaspoon salt
1 teaspoon lemon juice	

Place carrots and water in a saucepan, cover, and simmer 15 minutes, or until tender. Drain and pour carrots into a serving dish. Melt butter in the same saucepan; add parsley, lemon juice, and salt, stirring and heating through. Pour sauce over carrots and toss well. Serve at once.

Makes 4 servings

Glazed Carrots

GLUTEN-FREE
EGG-FREE

Never underestimate the power of orange juice, honey, and ginger to make something marvelous of the mundane! Use dairy-free margarine instead of butter, if you must.

1 pound slender fresh carrots
2 tablespoons butter
1 tablespoon honey
½ cup orange juice
½ teaspoon salt
¼ teaspoon ginger

Scrape carrots and cut into ¼-inch diagonal slices. Cook in a small amount of water, covered, 15–20 minutes, or until tender. Meanwhile, melt butter in a skillet; stir in honey and orange juice. Simmer 5 minutes. Stir in salt and ginger. Add cooked carrots, stirring carefully until they are completely glazed.

Makes 6 servings

Cucumber Yogurt Salad

GLUTEN-FREE
EGG-FREE

This dish has Middle Eastern origins. Great for a side dish on a hot summer day.

2 medium cucumbers, pared and sliced thin
1 teaspoon salt
2 tablespoons tarragon vinegar
1 tablespoon chopped fresh dillweed
1 cup plain yogurt
1 clove crushed garlic

Sprinkle cucumbers with salt and let stand for 20 minutes. Meanwhile, in a small bowl, mix vinegar, dillweed, yogurt, and crushed garlic; add to cucumbers and chill 1 hour before serving.

Makes 6 servings

Italian Greens

GLUTEN-FREE
EGG-FREE

Dark green leafy vegetables are good sources of calcium and vitamin A. Here's a way to turn ordinary greens into a delectable dish.

2 pounds fresh collard,   **¼ teaspoon sugar**
** kale, or turnip greens**   **⅛ teaspoon pepper**
1 clove garlic, crushed   **¼ cup grated Parmesan cheese**
1 tablespoon olive oil   **Raw onion rings**

Trim and wash greens. Mix garlic, oil, sugar, and pepper in a shallow saucepan; add trimmed greens and cover with a ½ inch water. Bring to a boil, cover, and reduce heat; cook until tender. Turn onto a serving plate and sprinkle with cheese. Top with raw onion rings.

Makes 6 servings

Dilled Peas

GLUTEN-FREE
EGG-FREE

Just a touch of herbs and a bit of butter (or dairy-free margarine) can lift frozen peas to a delectable height. Don't overcook those peas!

1 pound fresh peas *or* 1 10-ounce package frozen peas
1 small onion, chopped fine
1 tablespoon butter
½ teaspoon dried dillweed

Cook peas in water until tender, or steam them if preferred. Drain. Sauté onion in butter; add dillweed. Toss with drained peas and serve.

Makes 4 servings

Spinach-Stuffed Potatoes

GLUTEN-FREE

Baked potatoes are good for you, especially if you eat the mineral-laden skin. Here they combine with spinach to make a complete vegetable offering.

4 large baking potatoes
¾ cup cooked chopped
   spinach, well drained
½ cup grated Parmesan cheese
2 tablespoons grated onion
3 tablespoons milk
2 tablespoons butter
1 egg
1 teaspoon salt
⅛ teaspoon pepper

Scrub potatoes, dry, and prick with a fork. Bake in a 425° F. oven 1 hour, or until soft. Cut a slice from the top of each; carefully scoop out potato from skins. Place potato in a large bowl and mash well. Add spinach, cheese, onion, milk, butter, egg, salt, and pepper; beat well. Pile potato mixture back into the potato shells. Bake in a 350° F. oven for 25 minutes.

Makes 4 servings

Creamy Potato Salad

GLUTEN-FREE

Here's a delicious way to make potato salad. Sour cream lightens the texture of the dressing.

2 pounds potatoes, cooked, pared, and cooled
2 scallions, sliced thin
2 hard-cooked eggs, sliced thin
2 stalks celery, sliced thin
1 cup Mayonnaise (see recipe)
½ cup dairy sour cream
1 teaspoon salt
⅛ teaspoon pepper
2 tablespoons lemon juice

Cut potatoes into chunks and place in a large bowl. Add scallions, eggs, and celery; toss together. Combine mayonnaise, sour cream, salt, pepper, and lemon juice; mix thoroughly. Pour dressing over potatoes and toss lightly. Chill.

Makes 4–6 servings

Crustless Spinach Quiche

GLUTEN-FREE

When you can't have crust because of a gluten allergy, you can bake your quiche without it. Here's a firm combination that will hold together.

2 10-ounce packages frozen chopped spinach
1 cup ricotta cheese
¼ cup chopped scallions
1 egg, beaten
½ teaspoon salt
¼ teaspoon nutmeg

Cook spinach in a small amount of water until tender. Drain. Stir together ricotta cheese, scallions, egg, salt, and nutmeg; add cooked spinach. Pour into a greased 9-inch pie pan. Bake in a 350° F. oven for 25 minutes, or until firm. Serve hot.

Makes 6 servings

Spinach in Citrus Sauce

GLUTEN-FREE

Popeye would love this way of serving spinach! Use dairy-free margarine in place of butter, if necessary.

2 10-ounce packages frozen chopped spinach
1 egg yolk
1½ teaspoons lemon juice
¼ cup butter, melted and hot
2 tablespoons orange juice

Cook spinach as directed on the package. Meanwhile, place egg yolk and lemon juice in an electric blender (or food processor) container; cover and run on low speed. While blender is running, remove cover and add a thin stream of the hot melted butter. When all the butter has been blended, turn off blender. Stir in orange juice. Drain cooked spinach and fold sauce into it.

Makes 6 servings

Mashed Yellow Turnips

GLUTEN-FREE
EGG-FREE

If you don't have mace in your larder, use nutmeg instead— it's a close relative. Those who are dairy-sensitive should use dairy-free margarine instead of butter.

1½ pounds yellow turnips,
  peeled and cut up
4 tablespoons butter
½ teaspoon grated lemon rind

½ teaspoon salt
¼ teaspoon mace
⅛ teaspoon pepper

Cook turnips in a small amount of water for about 20 minutes, or until soft. Drain and mash. Add butter, lemon rind, salt, mace, and pepper, whipping well together.

Makes 4–6 servings

SAUCES

Blender Hollandaise

GLUTEN-FREE

Here's the easiest way to make Hollandaise Sauce. It will keep in the refrigerator for several days. Warm it by setting the jar in hot water.

¼ pound butter
2 eggs yolks

2 teaspoons lemon juice
¼ teaspoon salt

Melt butter in a small saucepan. Place egg yolks in an electric blender (or food processor); add lemon juice and salt. Blend on high and then turn to low. Add melted butter a little at a time. Turn blender off at the last drop, as mixture gets creamy and thick. Refrigerate in a tightly covered jar for several days to use as needed. To reheat, stand jar in simmering water after bringing to room temperature.

Makes 1 cup

Peanut Butter Curry Sauce

GLUTEN-FREE
EGG-FREE

Here's an interesting sauce to serve with chicken or to pour over a whole head of cooked cauliflower.

2 tablespoons butter
¼ cup finely chopped onion
1 medium apple, peeled,
   cored, and chopped
1 tablespoon cornstarch

1 tablespoon curry powder
½ teaspoon salt
1¼ cups milk
3 tablespoons creamy or
   chunky peanut butter

Melt butter in a small saucepan over medium heat. Add onion and apple; sauté until tender. Mix together cornstarch, curry powder, and salt. Gradually stir in milk until smooth. Add to apple mixture. Cook over medium heat, stirring constantly, until mixture comes to boil. Stir and boil for 1 minute. Add peanut butter, stirring until blended. Serve with cooked chicken.

Makes about 1¾ cups

Potato Starch White Sauce

GLUTEN-FREE/
EGG-FREE

If you have trouble finding potato starch flour, ask your health food store to obtain it for you. Sometimes it is labeled potato starch and sometimes potato flour, but it's the same thing.

2 tablespoons butter
2 tablespoons potato
   starch flour

1 cup milk
½ teaspoon salt

Melt butter in a saucepan; stir in flour until bubbling. Gradually stir in milk and add salt. Stir and cook until mixture thickens. (A thinner sauce may be made by reducing the amount of butter and potato starch flour to 1 tablespoon each. A thicker sauce may be made by increasing the amount of butter and potato starch flour to 3 tablespoons each.)

Makes about 1 cup

Cornstarch White Sauce Mix

GLUTEN-FREE/
EGG-FREE

Gluten-sensitive people will be happy to know that thickened sauces needn't be eliminated from their meals—make them with a cornstarch thickener. Here's how to do it!

2¾ cups instant nonfat dry milk
½ cup cornstarch
1 teaspoon salt
½ teaspoon pepper

Stir together dry milk, cornstarch, salt, and pepper. Store in a tightly covered container at room temperature. Stir this mix before each use.

Makes 2⅔ cups dry mix

Medium White Sauce

2 tablespoons butter
⅓ cup White Sauce Mix
¾ cup water

Melt butter in a small saucepan over low heat. Remove from heat; stir in White Sauce mix and water. Return to heat and bring to a boil, stirring constantly. Boil 1 minute. *Makes about 1 cup*

Thin White Sauce

Follow directions for Medium White Sauce, using ⅓ cup White Sauce Mix and 1 cup water. *Makes about 1 cup*

Thick White Sauce

Follow directions for Medium White Sauce, using ⅔ cup White Sauce Mix and 1 cup water. *Makes about 1 cup*

NOODLES, GRAINS, AND BREADS

Rice Flour Egg Noodles

GLUTEN-FREE
DAIRY-FREE

You can find rice noodles in an Oriental market, but you can also make them yourself. Be sure to let the dough rest between handling, as directed.

⅓ cup rice flour
½ teaspoon salt
½ teaspoon baking powder
2 egg yolks
1 scant tablespoon water

Combine rice flour, salt, and baking powder; place on a board and make a well in the center. Beat egg yolks and water together and pour into the well. Work flour mixture into the yolks until a soft dough forms. Sprinkle a little more rice flour on the board and knead the dough until pliable enough to roll out. Sprinkle board with a little more rice flour and roll dough thin. Let dry for about 15 minutes, then roll up and slice into fine noodles. Allow noodles to dry for at least 15 minutes more. Cook in boiling water or refrigerate in a plastic bag until ready to use. Keeps for 2–3 days.

Makes 4 servings, when added to soup

Mushroom Risotto

GLUTEN-FREE
EGG-FREE

Milk-sensitive diners can skip the cheese and use dairy-free margarine in place of butter and still have a very good rice dish.

3 tablespoons butter
1 cup uncooked rice
½ cup chopped onion
½ cup diced green pepper
1 cup sliced fresh mushrooms
2 cups Chicken Broth (see recipe)
1 teaspoon salt
½ cup grated Parmesan cheese

Melt butter in a large skillet; sauté rice until it glistens and becomes golden. Add onion, green pepper, and mushrooms. Continue cooking 5 minutes, stirring constantly to prevent overbrowning. Add chicken broth and salt. Bring to a boil and stir once. Cover, reduce heat, and simmer 15 minutes or until rice is tender and liquid is absorbed. Remove from heat. Toss lightly with cheese.

Makes 4–6 servings

Rice Flour Dumplings

GLUTEN-FREE
EGG-FREE

If dumplings are your thing, and you've been deprived because of a gluten sensitivity, here's the way to have them again.

1 cup rice flour
1½ teaspoons baking powder
¼ teaspoon salt
2 tablespoons rendered chicken fat or vegetable oil
½ cup milk
Chicken Broth (see recipe) or water

Sift rice flour, baking powder, and salt into a bowl. Stir in fat. Add milk and mix well. (If mixture is too thick to handle, add additional milk, a few teaspoons at a time.) Form mixture into 1-inch balls. Drop into boiling chicken broth or water. Cover and cook 12 minutes. Serve in soup or as an accompaniment to meat and vegetables.

Makes 4 servings

Gluten-Free Yeast Bread

GLUTEN-FREE

The gluten-sensitive yearn for anything that looks like a slice of bread. Gluten does have a quality that is not easily duplicated. But this yeast bread comes close!

1 pound cornstarch
½ cup nonfat dry milk
2 tablespoons sugar
2 teaspoons salt
½ cup milk
½ cup butter or margarine
¼ cup very warm water (approx. 110° F.)
1 package active dry yeast
3 eggs, beaten

Mix cornstarch, nonfat dry milk, sugar, and salt together. Scald milk; add butter or margarine and cool to lukewarm. Pour warm water into a large mixing bowl; sprinkle yeast over the water and stir until dissolved. Add milk-butter mixture and eggs to yeast mixture; blend well. Gradually add dry ingredients, stirring just until smooth. (Batter will be soft and shiny.) Cover. Let rise in a warm place, free of drafts, until double in bulk, about 1 hour. Stir down gently. Turn into a greased 9-by-5-inch loaf pan. Cover; let rise as before, until dough is 1 inch below the top of the pan, about 20 minutes. Bake in a 400° F. oven 20 minutes, then lower oven to 375° F. and continue baking until bread is golden brown, about 10 minutes more. Cool. Wrap and store in refrigerator.

Makes 1 loaf

Wheat-Free Banana Bread

GLUTEN-FREE

Bananas do have a very good effect on texture in a wheat-free bread. This batter bread will be a welcome treat.

1 cup rice flour	¼ cup sugar
1 tablespoon baking powder	2 eggs, separated
½ teaspoon salt	½ cup milk
¼ cup butter, softened	1 ripe banana, mashed

Sift together rice flour, baking powder, and salt; set aside. Cream butter; add sugar and beat until well blended. Beat in egg yolks. Add flour mixture alternately with milk, beating after each addition; add mashed banana. Beat egg whites until stiff peaks form and fold batter into egg whites. Spoon into a greased 9-by-5-inch loaf pan and bake in a preheated 325° F. oven for 45 minutes. Cool before slicing.

Makes 1 loaf

Wheat-Free Banana Nut Bread

GLUTEN-FREE
DAIRY-FREE

Here's a banana bread that is both gluten-free and dairy-free for those with double problems. And it's delicious!

1½ cups rice flour
1 cup potato starch
1 tablespoon baking powder
1⅓ cups mashed banana
¼ cup light brown sugar
½ teaspoon salt
2 eggs, beaten
½ cup salad oil
2 tablespoons water
¼ cup coarsely chopped walnuts

Sift together rice flour, potato starch, and baking powder. In a separate bowl, combine mashed banana, sugar, and salt; add beaten eggs, salad oil, and water. Mix well. Stir in dry ingredients. Add nuts. Pour into a greased 8-by-4-inch loaf pan. Let stand at room temperature for 5 minutes before placing in a preheated 350° F. oven. Bake for 1 hour. Transfer from pan onto a rack to cool.

Makes 8 servings

Rice Flour Herb Bread

GLUTEN-FREE

Batter breads are easy to stir and bake—a wonderful reason to enjoy them.

2 cups rice flour
¼ cup potato starch
½ cup nonfat dry milk solids
3 tablespoons baking powder
2 tablespoons chopped parsley
2 tablespoons chopped chives
1 tablespoon sugar
1 teaspoon salt
2 eggs
⅓ cup salad oil
2 tablespoons water

Combine rice flour, potato starch, dry milk solids, baking powder, parsley, chives, sugar, and salt. Beat eggs, oil, and water together; add to dry mixture and stir until just blended. Pour into a greased 8-by-3½-inch loaf pan. Let stand for 5 minutes before placing in a preheated 350° F. oven. Bake for 1 hour. Remove from pan and cool on a rack. This bread can be stored in a plastic bag in the refrigerator for several days.

Makes 16 slices

Gluten-Free Corn Bread

GLUTEN-FREE

Most corn breads have some wheat flour in the recipe, but this one is made from pure cornmeal and is mighty good. For a change of pace, add drained corn niblets to the batter!

2 cups cornmeal
1 tablespoon baking powder
2 tablespoons sugar
1 teaspoon salt
1 egg
1 cup milk
¼ cup corn oil

Combine cornmeal, baking powder, sugar, and salt. Beat egg in a bowl; add milk and corn oil and beat well. Gradually beat in the dry ingredients. Pour into a greased 9-by-9-by-2-inch pan. Bake in a preheated 375° F. oven for 25 minutes.

Makes 9 3-inch squares

Blueberry-Rice Muffins

GLUTEN-FREE
EGG-FREE

Because of the gluten factor in wheat and related grains, it is sometimes disappointing to bake with nongluten flour because the results are less spongy. Muffins are a better choice. Butter in this recipe can be exchanged for dairy-free margarine, if desired.

1½ cups rice flour
⅔ cup hot water
2 tablespoons butter
¼ cup sugar
3 tablespoons baking powder
¼ teaspoon salt
1 teaspoon vanilla
1 teaspoon grated lemon rind
½ cup fresh blueberries,
  washed, stems removed

Combine half the flour with the hot water; set aside. Cream together butter and sugar; add flour mixture and beat well. Stir together remaining flour, sugar, baking powder, and salt and add flour mixture, vanilla, and grated lemon rind to batter. Stir in blueberries. Spoon into a greased muffin tin and bake in a 375° F. oven for 20 minutes.

Makes 8

Banana Rice Flour Biscuits

GLUTEN-FREE
EGG-FREE

Once again, a ripe banana comes to the rescue when using rice flour. Extra biscuits may be frozen for future meals.

1 cup rice flour
2 teaspoons baking powder
¼ teaspoon salt
1½ teaspoons sugar
2 tablespoons butter, softened
½ cup mashed ripe banana
⅓ cup milk

Combine rice flour, baking powder, salt, and sugar. Add butter and cut in until mixture resembles meal. Add banana and milk; mix thoroughly. Form into a cylinder and cut biscuits. Place on a greased cookie sheet touching each other. Bake in a preheated 400° F. oven for 20–25 minutes, or until lightly browned.

Makes 8

Onion Potato Flour Muffins

GLUTEN-FREE
DAIRY-FREE

Beat the egg whites until really stiff to get a nice tall muffin. Grease with oil instead of butter to keep the recipe dairy-free.

4 eggs, separated
1 tablespoon sugar
¼ teaspoon salt
2 tablespoons cold water

½ cup potato flour
1 teaspoon baking powder
½ teaspoon powdered onion

Beat egg yolks until lemon-colored. Add sugar, salt, and cold water. Sift together potato flour, baking powder, and powdered onion; add gradually to egg yolks. Beat egg whites until stiff peaks form; fold into batter. Bake in a greased muffin tin in a preheated 350° F. oven for 15–20 minutes, or until lightly browned.

Makes 8

DESSERTS

Lemon Cups

GLUTEN-FREE

A delicate pudding is the perfect ending for a routine meal. Here's a shimmering cup of lemon fluff that's pure delight.

1 cup sugar
¼ cup rice flour
2 tablespoons vegetable oil
Dash of salt

2 teaspoons grated lemon peel
⅓ cup lemon juice
1½ cups milk, scalded
3 eggs, separated

Combine sugar, rice flour, oil, and salt. Add lemon peel and juice. Stir milk into egg yolks; beat well and add to lemon mixture. Beat egg whites stiff; fold into lemon mixture. Pour into 8 ungreased 5-ounce custard cups. Set cups into a shallow pan; pour hot water around them, 1-inch deep. Bake at 325° F. for 40 minutes, or until cake part (atop the sauce) is done. Serve warm or chilled.

Makes 8 servings

Chocolate-Vanilla Parfaits

GLUTEN-FREE

It's so easy to create a glamorous dessert when you have a few minutes to putter in the morning. Chill for later.

2 envelopes unflavored gelatin
1½ cups cold milk
1 cup boiling milk
2 eggs
⅓ cup sugar
⅛ teaspoon salt
2 teaspoons pure vanilla extract
6 ice cubes
¼ cup sugar
3 tablespoons unsweetened pure cocoa

Sprinkle gelatin over ½ cup of the cold milk in an electric blender (or food processor) container. Add boiling milk; cover and blend on high speed until gelatin is dissolved. Add the eggs, the ⅓ cup sugar, the salt, 1 teaspoon of the vanilla, and the remaining 1 cup cold milk. Cover and blend until smooth. While blender is running, add ice cubes, one at a time. Continue blending until ice is dissolved. Spoon half of the mixture (about 2 cups) from blender container into a bowl and stir in the remaining 1 teaspoon vanilla; set aside. Add the ¼ cup sugar and the cocoa to the mixture remaining in the blender container; cover and blend until smooth. Layer chocolate and vanilla mixtures in tall glasses. Chill at least 2 hours, or until set.

Makes 6–8 servings

Orange Parfaits

GLUTEN-FREE

This recipe can easily be divided in half. Use the remainder of the concentrate for breakfast juice.

2 envelopes unflavored gelatin
½ cup cold water
½ cup boiling water
2 eggs
⅔ cup sugar
⅛ teaspoon salt
1 6-ounce can frozen orange juice concentrate
1 cup heavy cream
6 ice cubes

Sprinkle gelatin over cold water in a blender container. Add boiling water; cover and blend on low speed until gelatin is dissolved. Add eggs, sugar, and salt; cover and blend on high speed. Add heavy cream and ice cubes, one at a time. Continue blending until ice is dissolved. Pour into parfait glasses. Chill 1 hour.

Makes 8 servings

Custard Fruit Cup

GLUTEN-FREE

Use this custard when you are able to buy fresh berries. It makes a delectable creation!

4 eggs
½ cup sugar
¼ teaspoon salt
2½ cups milk, scalded
1½ teaspoons pure vanilla extract
3 cups cut-up fresh fruit

Beat eggs; add sugar and salt. Gradually pour scalded milk

into the egg mixture, stirring constantly. Cook in the top of a double boiler over simmering water, stirring constantly, until mixture coats a metal spoon. Stir in vanilla. Cool immediately. Cover with foil, plastic wrap, or waxed paper and refrigerate. To serve, put ½ cup fresh fruit in each dessert dish. Spoon ½ cup custard over fruit. Garnish with a few additional pieces of fresh fruit before serving.

Makes 6 servings

Baked Rice Pudding

GLUTEN-FREE
EGG-FREE

This is an old-fashioned way of baking a simple rice pudding. Add a handful of seedless raisins to perk it up.

½ cup white rice
1 quart milk
¼ cup sugar
⅛ teaspoon salt
1 teaspoon pure vanilla extract
Whipped cream (optional)

Preheat oven to 325° F. Combine rice, milk, sugar, salt, and vanilla. Pour into a buttered casserole; cover. Bake about 2 hours, or until rice has softened. Remove cover and bake a few minutes longer. Serve with whipped cream, if desired.

Makes 8 servings

Rice Cream with Honeyed Fig Topping

GLUTEN-FREE

This is definitely company fare. Serve molded desserts on tall, pedestaled platters for the utmost gourmet effect.

1 envelope unflavored gelatin
1½ cups milk
1 3-ounce package cream cheese, softened
2 eggs, separated
¼ cup sugar
1 cup cooked rice
1 teaspoon pure vanilla extract
1 recipe Honeyed Fig Topping (below)

Soften gelatin in ½ cup of the milk; set aside. In a large saucepan, blend the remaining 1 cup milk with cream cheese. Beat egg yolks slightly and stir into the cream cheese mixture with half of the sugar. Stir in the gelatin mixture. Cook over low heat, stirring constantly, until mixture coats a spoon. Stir in rice and vanilla. Cool slightly. Beat egg whites until frothy; then gradually beat in the remaining sugar, beating until whites are stiff. Gently fold into the rice mixture. Turn into a 1-quart mold. Chill until firm. Unmold and cut into wedges; serve with Honeyed Fig Topping (below).

Makes 6–8 servings

Honeyed Fig Topping

GLUTEN-FREE

1 cup dried figs   2 tablespoons honey
3 tablespoons lemon juice

Put dried figs through a food grinder. Mix with lemon juice and honey. Cover tightly and refrigerate about 24 hours or until fruit softens and flavors blend.

Makes 1¼ cups

Creamy Rice Mold

GLUTEN-FREE

Plan to cook extra rice for dinner so you'll have leftovers for next day's dessert. Egg whites are stiff when they can be pulled into firm peaks.

1 1-tablespoon envelope unflavored gelatin
1½ cups milk
1 3-ounce package cream cheese, softened
2 eggs, separated
1 tablespoon sugar
1 cup cooked rice
1 teaspoon pure vanilla extract

Soften gelatin in ½ cup milk. Blend remaining milk with cream cheese. Stir in lightly beaten egg yolks and half of the sugar. Add gelatin. Cook over low heat, stirring constantly, until mixture coats a spoon. Add rice and vanilla; cool slightly. Beat egg whites until frothy, then gradually beat in the remaining sugar and continue beating until whites are stiff. Gently fold into rice mixture. Turn into a 1-quart mold. Chill until firm. Cut into wedges and serve with fresh berries or other fruit.

Makes 6–8 servings

Lemon Chiffon Dessert

GLUTEN-FREE

Buy some fancy-shaped molds and use them for these intriguing desserts. It makes them look very special.

1 1-tablespoon envelope unflavored gelatin
2 tablespoons sugar
⅛ teaspoon salt
2 eggs, separated
2 cups milk
2 teaspoons grated lemon rind
2 tablespoons lemon juice
2 tablespoons sugar

Mix together gelatin, 2 tablespoons sugar, and salt in a saucepan. Beat egg yolks in a bowl; add milk and stir into gelatin mixture. Place over very low heat, stirring constantly, until gelatin dissolves and mixture thickens slightly, about 5 minutes. Remove from heat. Stir in grated lemon rind and lemon juice. Chill, stirring occasionally, until mixture is thickened but not lumpy (until it mounds slightly when dropped from a spoon). Beat egg whites until soft peaks form; gradually add 2 tablespoons sugar and beat until stiff. Fold gelatin mixture into beaten egg whites. Turn into a 4-cup bowl or mold or into 4 individual 1-cup serving dishes. Chill until set.

Makes 6 servings

Baked Fresh Pears

GLUTEN-FREE
EGG-FREE

Exchange dairy-free margarine for the butter and you can serve this to the milk-sensitive person, who will feel no deprivation!

3 firm fresh pears, pared,
   halved, and cored
2 tablespoons fresh lemon juice
2 tablespoons butter

6 tablespoons pure maple
   syrup
½ cup boiling water

Brush pears with lemon juice. Arrange in a shallow baking dish. Place 1 teaspoon butter and 1½ teaspoons maple syrup in each pear half. Mix remaining 3 tablespoons maple syrup with boiling water and pour into the bottom of the baking dish. Bake uncovered in a 400° F. oven for 1 hour, or until tender, basting occasionally with pan liquid. Serve as a dessert or as a side dish with meats or poultry.

Makes 6 servings

Blueberry Delight

GLUTEN-FREE
EGG-FREE

Spoon delicately flavored lemon yogurt on top of fresh berries to give a festive air to this dessert.

1 pint fresh blueberries, chilled
½ cup lemon natural yogurt
1 teaspoon grated fresh lemon rind

Wash, drain, and pick over the berries, discarding all stems, leaves, and berries of poor quality. Fill 4 sherbet glasses with the berries. Top with a generous dollop of lemon yogurt. Sprinkle with grated lemon rind.

Makes 4 servings

Ricotta Rice Cheescake

GLUTEN-FREE

You'll be unaware of the rice when this cake is served, but it does play a role in holding things together. A winning cake!

3 eggs
1½ cups sugar
1½ cups ricotta cheese
½ cup milk
2 teaspoons grated lemon peel
5 cups cooked rice

Beat together eggs and sugar for 1 minute. Mash cheese slightly and mix with milk and lemon peel; add to egg mixture. Beat until smooth. Stir in cooked rice. Pour into a buttered 9-inch square baking dish. Bake at 350° F. for 1 hour. Serve warm.

Makes 9 servings

Refrigerator Cherry Cheesecake

GLUTEN-FREE

Here's one of the best no-bake cheesecakes ever devised. If desired, fresh pitted cherries may be used for the topping— spoon melted currant jelly over the top for a glazed effect.

1 cup skim milk
4 eggs
2 1-tablespoon envelopes unflavored gelatin
1 cup sugar
1 teaspoon pure vanilla
2 pounds cream-style cottage cheese, sieved
1 14½-ounce jar pitted dark sweet cherries
1 teaspoon cornstarch

Pour milk into the top of a double boiler. Beat in eggs. Mix gelatin and sugar together; stir into the milk mixture. Cook over boiling water, stirring constantly, until gelatin is dissolved and mixture has thickened, 10–15 minutes. Remove from heat and cool slightly. Stir vanilla into sieved cottage cheese, then stir in cooled gelatin mixture. Pour into an 8-inch springform pan. Chill until almost firm. Drain syrup from jar of dark sweet cherries into a saucepan. Stir in cornstarch. Bring to a boil, stirring constantly. Cook 1 minute longer. Arrange drained cherries on top of cheesecake. Spoon ⅓ cup of thickened syrup over cherries. Chill until firm. Rest of syrup may be spooned over portions of cheesecake at serving time, if desired.

Makes 12 servings

English Sponge Cake

GLUTEN-FREE
DAIRY-FREE

You can have your cake despite a wheat allergy! Here's the way to do it. Be sure to invert the pans as soon as they leave the oven so the sponge stays tall.

1 cup sifted confectioners' sugar
⅔ cup sifted cornstarch
3 eggs, separated
2 tablespoons water
⅛ teaspoon cream of tartar
½ teaspoon vanilla extract

Sift ½ cup of the sugar and all of the cornstarch, then sift again. Beat egg whites, water, and cream of tartar in a large mixing bowl, until very soft peaks form. Gradually beat in remaining ½ cup sugar, beating until stiff peaks form. Add egg yolks and vanilla; beat just until blended. Sift cornstarch mixture a little at a time over egg mixture, folding until well blended after each addition. Turn into two ungreased 8-inch round cake pans. Bake in a 350° F. oven 25–30 minutes, or until cake springs back when touched. Remove from oven and invert on wire racks. Cool completely.

Makes 2 8-inch layers

Rice Flour Sponge Cake

GLUTEN-FREE
DAIRY-FREE

Just in case there's a sensitivity to corn, here's a way to make a sponge cake with rice flour. The secret of a firm sponge cake is to beat those egg whites until they stand up and form stiff peaks.

4 eggs, separated
⅔ cup sugar
¼ teaspoon salt
2 tablespoons lemon juice
Grated rind of ½ lemon
1 cup rice flour

Beat egg yolks until thick and lemon-colored. Add sugar and salt and beat well. Add lemon juice and grated lemon rind. Gradually add rice flour and beat until smooth. Let batter stand for about 10 minutes. Then beat egg whites until stiff peaks form. Fold beaten whites into the batter. Pour into an ungreased 9-inch tube pan. Bake in a preheated 350° F. oven for 50–60 minutes, or until lightly browned and firm. Invert immediately after removing from oven and cool completely.

Makes 12 servings

Lemon Sponge Cake

GLUTEN-FREE
DAIRY-FREE

If there's a corn and rice sensitivity, make the sponge cake with potato flour. Flip it upside down immediately upon taking out of the oven so it doesn't fall.

6 eggs, separated   **1 cup sifted potato flour**
1 whole egg   **½ teaspoon salt**
1½ cups sugar   **½ teaspoon nutmeg**
2 tablespoons lemon juice **Confectioners' sugar**
Grated rind of 1 lemon   **(optional)**

Preheat oven to 350° F. Beat egg yolks and whole egg together until foamy; beat in sugar and add lemon juice and rind. Sift together potato flour and salt; add to egg yolk batter with nutmeg. Beat egg whites until stiff and fold into the batter. Grease the bottom of a 10-inch springform pan and pour batter into the pan. Bake 35 minutes, or until the cake is firm in the center. Cool upside down before removing the sides of the springform pan. Dust with confectioners' sugar, if desired.

Makes 12 servings

Orange Sponge Cake

GLUTEN-FREE
DAIRY-FREE

If you have a supply of millet flour (a European grain that is sold in health food stores), here's an orange-flavored sponge cake to make with it.

4 eggs, separated
1 cup sugar
¼ cup orange juice
1 cup ground millet flour
2 teaspoons baking powder

Beat egg yolks until lemon-colored. Add sugar and beat well. Add orange juice. Add millet flour and baking powder, mixing well. Beat egg whites until stiff peaks form. Carefully fold egg whites into batter until completely blended but spongy with air bubbles. Pour into an ungreased 9-inch tube pan and bake in a preheated 350° F. oven for 30 minutes, or until top is browned and firm to the touch. Immediately upon removing from oven, invert tube pan onto a cake rack or onto the neck of an empty soda bottle. Allow cake to cool completely in this upside-down position.

Makes 10–12 servings

Vanilla Cupcakes

GLUTEN-FREE

Cleaning muffin pans is easier if you poke a fluted paper muffin holder into each ungreased cup, then fill and bake. The muffins look prettier too!

⅓ cup butter	1 cup sifted cornstarch
⅓ cup sugar	1 teaspoon baking powder
1 egg	3 tablespoons milk
¼ teaspoon pure vanilla extract	

Preheat oven to 375° F. Cream butter and sugar together; add egg and vanilla. Sift together cornstarch and baking powder and add to the batter alternately with the milk. Spoon the batter into a greased muffin tin, filling ⅔ full. Bake 12–15 minutes, or until a toothpick inserted in the center of a cupcake comes out clean.

Makes 8 servings

Chocolate Mounds

GLUTEN-FREE
DAIRY-FREE

There's no sense in feeling deprived of goodies just because there's an allergy to wheat. Here's a nice mouthful of chocolate that all will enjoy.

¼ cup cornstarch
½ teaspoon ground cinnamon
¼ teaspoon baking powder
¼ teaspoon salt
6 1-ounce squares semisweet chocolate
2 1-ounce squares unsweetened chocolate
2 tablespoons margarine
2 eggs
¾ cup firmly packed brown sugar
1 6-ounce package semisweet chocolate pieces
2 cups coarsely chopped walnuts or pecans

In a medium bowl, stir together cornstarch, cinnamon, baking powder, and salt. In a small saucepan, melt chocolate and margarine over very low heat. In a large bowl, beat eggs and sugar until thick and glossy. Gradually add chocolate mixture to egg mixture, stirring until smooth. Stir in cornstarch mixture just until moistened. Stir in chocolate pieces and nuts. Drop batter by heaping teaspoonfuls 1 inch apart onto an ungreased cookie sheet. Bake in a 350° F. oven 10–12 minutes, or until cookies are firm on the outside. Do not overbake. Cool on a wire rack.

Makes about 3½ dozen

NOTE: If keeping cookies more than 2 days, store in freezer.

Cocoa Almond Meringue Cookies

GLUTEN-FREE
DAIRY-FREE

The secret of meringue cookies is the low oven temperature. Pay attention to that, and you'll enjoy the results.

¾ **cup sugar, divided**
⅓ **cup blanched almonds, ground fine**
2 **tablespoons sifted cornstarch**
3 **tablespoons sifted unsweetened cocoa**
3 **egg whites**
⅛ **teaspoon cream of tartar**
Dash of salt
½ **teaspoon vanilla extract**

Line cookie sheets with wax paper or foil. In a small bowl, stir together ¼ cup of the sugar, the almonds, cornstarch, and cocoa. In a large bowl with a mixer at high speed, beat the egg whites until foamy; add cream of tartar and salt. Continue beating until soft peaks form. Gradually add the remaining ½ cup sugar; beat until stiff peaks form. Add vanilla. Fold in almond mixture. Spoon onto cookie sheet to form 1½-inch rounds. Bake in a 325° F. oven 20 minutes, or until dry. Remove and cool on wire racks.

Makes about 3 dozen

Macaroons

Almonds can be ground in a blender or food processor in just a moment or two. Don't forget to cover the cookie sheet with aluminum foil!

1¼ cups ground blanched almonds
¾ cup sugar
2 egg whites
2 tablespoons cornstarch
2 teaspoons water
¼ teaspoon pure vanilla extract
18–20 blanched almond halves

Combine ground almonds and sugar. Add unbeaten egg whites, reserving about 1 tablespoon to brush on top of macaroons. Stir for 1 minute, or until well blended. Add cornstarch, water, and vanilla, stirring well after each addition. Drop batter 3 inches apart onto foil-covered baking sheet by teaspoonfuls. Brush cookies with remaining egg white, then place an almond half on top of each. Bake in 375° F. oven 15 minutes, or until evenly browned. Cool on a wire rack 3–4 minutes, or until foil may be peeled off. Remove foil; cool cookies on a wire rack.

Makes about 1½ dozen

Chewy Crisps

There are so many ways to eat peanut butter. Here's an easy way to bake it into delectable cookies!

1 cup creamy or chunky peanut butter
1 cup sugar
½ cup undiluted evaporated milk
4 teaspoons cornstarch

Mix together peanut butter, sugar, milk, and cornstarch. Drop by teaspoonfuls onto an ungreased baking sheet. Bake in a 350° F. oven 12–15 minutes, or until light golden brown. Cool 1–2 minutes before removing from baking sheet.

Makes 36

Date-Nut Cookies

GLUTEN-FREE
DAIRY-FREE

If you like your cookies crunchy and filled with fruit and coconut, you're going to enjoy these very much. Don't forget to chill the dough.

2 eggs
½ cup light brown sugar
1 teaspoon vanilla extract
½ teaspoon salt
¾ cup creamy or chunky peanut butter
½ cup chopped dates
½ cup flaked coconut

Beat the eggs in a mixing bowl with a rotary beater until thick and lemon-colored. Stir in sugar, vanilla, and salt. Add peanut butter, dates, and coconut; mix well. Chill 2–3 hours. Drop by teaspoonfuls onto a greased cookie sheet. Flatten with a fork, making a crosshatch pattern on each. Bake in a 300° F. oven until cookies are lightly browned, about 25 minutes.

Makes 2½ dozen

7
How to Deal with Multiple Allergies

Many people have multiple allergies and must eliminate all dairy products, eggs, and gluten flours (made from wheat, rye, oats, and barley) from their diets. This is the most difficult of all restrictions for planning menus and maintaining good health. If you have patience and determination, however, you can still eat nutritious and flavorful meals.

First, read the information at the beginning of chapters 4, 5, and 6 to build your knowledge of the three sensitivities discussed in this book. Then get into the habit of writing down menus for at least one day, preferably for an entire week. This is the only way you can determine whether you are getting all the nutrients that the human body requires in order to function, grow, and develop at optimum levels.

It's important to understand that the human body is not an unchangeable entity—like a finished work of art—when it has matured to adulthood. Instead it is an ever-changing group of cells that require nurturing in order to maintain good health. Bones are constantly breaking down and rebuilding cells, teeth are not as solid as cement but rather are also in a state of constant regrowth, and gums need to be fed sufficient vitamin C to hold those teeth in place.

Habits such as smoking and drinking alcoholic beverages rob the body of vitamins B and C, leaving you with insufficient supplies of these important nutrients unless they are replaced.

When you are planning a daily menu, be sure that you include plenty of fresh fruits and vegetables, including citrus fruits, to obtain your ration of vitamin C. Also be sure to eat at least one dark yellow or dark green vegetable a day to get vitamin A. Add whole brown rice and permissible baked goods to get vitamin B. These will also give you a good amount of complex carbohydrates and fiber.

Use one teaspoonful of oil on your salad to get your daily ration of vitamin E, which provides the essential fatty acids in the diet. If you do not get any sunshine during the day, you might want to consider taking some fish oil supplement to ensure your intake of vitamin D. Add meat, poultry, and fish to the menu so that at least 12 percent of your caloric intake is in high-protein foods. By using this menu planning system, you will safely be able to eliminate the three major food ingredients of dairy products, eggs, and gluten flour.

The recipes in this chapter may be used by those who have an allergy to any one of these foods, but they are designed to assist those who seem to be sensitive to all three categories and who understandably suffer confusion—and sometimes even malnutrition.

BEVERAGES

Orange Grape Punch

DAIRY-FREE
EGG-FREE
GLUTEN-FREE

Here's a refreshing fruit punch that has a kick of cinnamon. And it's better than a chemical-laden soda pop.

1 quart orange juice
1 quart grape juice

¼ teaspoon ground cinnamon
1 pint club soda

Combine orange juice, grape juice, and cinnamon. Refrigerate until ready to serve. Add club soda just before serving to preserve carbonation.

Makes 10 servings

Fruit Punch

DAIRY-FREE
EGG-FREE
GLUTEN-FREE

This makes a gallon of good drinking. Highly nutritious, too.

1 quart unsweetened pineapple juice
1 quart orange juice
1 quart unsweetened apple juice
1 quart unsweetened grape juice

Combine all juices and refrigerate until ready to serve. Pour into a punch bowl filled with a ring of ice. If carbonation is desired, add a small bottle of club soda just before serving.

Makes 16 servings

Grape Juice Sangria

DAIRY-FREE
EGG-FREE
GLUTEN-FREE

Make a nonalcoholic sangria with grape juice and fruit. Keep chilled until ready to serve.

1 quart unsweetened grape juice
1 pint unsweetened pineapple juice
1 orange, sliced thin
1 apple, cut into wedges
1 pint club soda

Combine grape juice, pineapple juice, sliced orange (with rind intact), and apple wedges. Let stand in refrigerator until ready to serve. At serving time, add club soda and pour over ice cubes. Be sure that each glass has some pieces of fruit in it.

Makes 8 servings

Spicy Apple Drink

DAIRY-FREE
EGG-FREE
GLUTEN-FREE

This is a perfect drink for chilly fall evenings when thoughts are on pumpkins and perhaps goblins, too!

1 quart unsweetened apple juice
1 teaspoon whole cloves
1 cinnamon stick
4 lemon slices

Heat apple juice with cloves and cinnamon stick. Remove these spices and pour juice into mugs, each containing a slice of lemon.

Makes 4 servings

Orange Pineapple Punch

DAIRY-FREE
EGG-FREE
GLUTEN-FREE

When you want to serve a natural fruit drink with no added sugar or artificial coloring or flavoring, here's a delicious combination to consider.

1 pint unsweetened pineapple juice
1 quart fresh orange juice
Juice of 1 lemon
1 quart club soda

Combine all ingredients (juices first) just before serving time.

Makes 10 servings

Ginger Grapefruit Drink

DAIRY-FREE
EGG-FREE
GLUTEN-FREE

If you prefer a tart and tangy taste, here's the drink that will hit the spot. Don't forget the ginger—it's the flavor enhancer!

1 quart grapefruit juice
1 quart club soda
1 teaspoon ground ginger
Mint leaves

Combine grapefruit juice, club soda, and ground ginger; stir well. Serve in chilled tall glasses with a sprig of mint.

Makes 8 servings

Tomato Cocktail

DAIRY-FREE
EGG-FREE
GLUTEN-FREE

Here's a trick to make tomato juice better. Add a celery stalk as a swizzle stick, if desired.

1 20-ounce can tomato juice
2 tablespoons lemon juice
¼ teaspoon celery salt
1 teaspoon Worcestershire sauce

Combine ingredients. Chill or serve over crushed ice.

Makes 4 servings

Hot Cider

DAIRY-FREE
EGG-FREE
GLUTEN-FREE

Want to give your apple cider a bit of a lift? This is the way to serve it hot and pungent.

2 quarts apple cider
Rind of 1 lemon
2 teaspoons Angostura bitters
1 orange, sliced thin

Combine apple cider, lemon rind, and Angostura bitters in a saucepan. Bring to a boil, lower heat, and simmer for 15 minutes. Remove lemon rind. Serve hot with a thin slice of orange floating in each glass.

Makes 8 servings

APPETIZERS

Fresh Fruit Compote

DAIRY-FREE
EGG-FREE
GLUTEN-FREE

Sometimes just the simplest combination of fruits can start a meal right. Chill for several hours to "marry" the flavors.

4 ripe bananas
2 cups fresh pineapple chunks
2 cups red grapes, halved and seeded
½ cup orange juice
2 teaspoons honey

Peel bananas and slice in chunks; place in a large bowl. Add pineapple chunks, grapes, orange juice, and honey. Toss to mix well. Cover and refrigerate until ready to serve.

Makes 8 servings

Fresh Fruit Salad

DAIRY-FREE
EGG-FREE
GLUTEN-FREE

Shredded coconut has a way of making things festive. Vary the fruit with the season.

3 grapefruits
3 oranges
1 cup fresh strawberries, sliced
¼ cup flaked coconut
Mint leaves

Chill grapefruits and oranges before preparing. Cut a slice from the top of each, then cut off peel in strips from top to bottom, cutting deep enough to remove white membrane. Then cut a slice from the bottom of each. Go over the fruit again, removing any remaining white membrane. Section the grapefruits and oranges. Add the strawberries. Turn into a serving bowl or individual dishes and sprinkle with coconut. Garnish with mint.

Makes 6–8 servings

Chopped Eggplant

DAIRY-FREE
EGG-FREE
GLUTEN-FREE

When there are multiple allergies it sometimes seems as if there's nothing to serve as a spread. Not true! Here's a recipe you'll use again and again.

1 whole eggplant (about 1 pound)
1 medium onion, sliced
1 medium green pepper, cut up
1 tablespoon olive oil
½ teaspoon salt
⅛ teaspoon pepper
1 tablespoon lemon juice

Bake the whole eggplant in a 350° F. oven until the skin is soft and wrinkled (approximately 20 minutes). Remove from oven and cut skin away. Chop in a large chopping bowl. Add onion and green pepper and chop all very fine. Add oil, salt, pepper, and lemon juice. Serve chilled on lettuce as an appetizer, or serve with crackers as a spread.

Makes about 2 cups

Pickled Mushrooms

DAIRY-FREE
EGG-FREE
GLUTEN-FREE

If you have a jar of these pickled mushrooms in the refrigerator, those with allergies will never feel deprived of an elegant appetizer.

1 pound fresh button mushrooms	1 clove garlic, minced fine
Salted boiling water	1 teaspoon grated onion
½ cup salad oil	½ teaspoon paprika
⅓ cup vinegar	½ teaspoon dry mustard
	2 whole cloves

Wash mushrooms and cut stems off even with the bottom of each mushroom; reserve stems for another use. Drop into boiling salted water and boil for about 3 minutes. Drain well. Combine salad oil, vinegar, garlic, onion, paprika, mustard, and cloves; pour over mushrooms. Cover and refrigerate at least a day before serving. May be kept for 1 week. Serve with toothpicks.

Makes 8–10 servings

Scampi

DAIRY-FREE
EGG-FREE
GLUTEN-FREE

This is a fast and tasty appetizer. May also be served as a main course to four lucky people!

¼ cup olive oil
2 cloves garlic, minced
1 pound shrimp, shelled and cleaned
¼ cup chopped parsley

Heat olive oil in a large skillet. Add minced garlic and brown lightly. Add shrimp and sauté until bright pink, about 4 minutes. Sprinkle parsley over all and mix well. Serve hot with toothpicks or fancy spears.

Makes 6 to 8 servings

SOUPS

Chicken Broth

DAIRY-FREE
EGG-FREE
GLUTEN-FREE

The secret of good chicken soup is to load it with herbs and then slip a teaspoon of sugar into the pot just before serving. Try it!

1 stewing chicken (a fowl), about 4 pounds
2 quarts water
1 whole onion, peeled
3 carrots, scraped
4 stalks celery, including tops
1 parsnip root, cleaned
2 sprigs parsley
2 sprigs dillweed
2 teaspoons salt
¼ teaspoon pepper
1 teaspoon sugar

Clean chicken, place in a deep pot, and add water and the remaining ingredients. Bring to a boil, then turn heat down and simmer, covered, until the chicken is tender, about 2 hours. Remove chicken, strain soup (saving a carrot), and chill. Skim off fat that solidifies. Reheat soup. Add sugar. Add additional salt and pepper, if desired. Serve with a piece of soup carrot in each bowl and with cooked noodles, if desired.

Makes 8 servings

Vegetable Soup

DAIRY-FREE
EGG-FREE
GLUTEN-FREE

Vegetable soup should be open-ended to include any leftover raw vegetables that are on hand. Be adventurous!

2 pounds beef neck bones
2 quarts water
2 onions, diced
2 carrots, scraped and diced
2 stalks celery, diced
1 teaspoon salt
¼ teaspoon pepper
1 pound lima beans, soaked for several hours
1 potato, peeled and diced
1 1-pound can tomatoes in natural juice
1 10-ounce package frozen cut green beans
1 10-ounce package frozen peas

Place bones and water in a deep pot. Bring to a boil, then simmer for 30 minutes. Skim residue from the top with a spoon. Add onions, carrots, celery, salt, and pepper. Simmer, covered, for 1 hour. Add soaked lima beans and simmer for 30 minutes. Add potato, tomatoes, green beans, and peas. Simmer 30 minutes more. Taste and add additional salt and pepper if needed.

Makes 8 servings

Carrot Soup

DAIRY-FREE
EGG-FREE
GLUTEN-FREE

In Europe carrot soup is considered the most soothing food for an upset stomach. It's mighty good when you're feeling fine, too!

8 carrots, sliced thin
1 onion, sliced thin
1 stalk celery, sliced thin
1 sprig parsley

1 quart water
½ teaspoon salt
⅛ teaspoon pepper
1 bay leaf

Place carrots, onion, celery, and parsley in a heavy saucepan. Add water, salt, pepper, and bay leaf. Bring to a boil, cover, and reduce heat to a simmer. Cook for 45 minutes, or until vegetables are soft enough to put through a sieve. Remove bay leaf. Put vegetables and soup through a sieve, or process in an electric blender or a food processor. Serve hot.

Makes 4–6 servings

Yellow Pea Soup

DAIRY-FREE
EGG-FREE
GLUTEN-FREE

If no veal bones are available, a ham bone or beef bone will do.

1¾ cups dried yellow peas
6 cups water
1 large onion, sliced thin
2 potatoes, peeled and quartered
2 or 3 veal bones with clinging meat
½ teaspoon salt
¼ teaspoon pepper

Place dried peas, water, onion, potatoes, bones, salt, and pepper in a deep saucepan. Bring to a boil, then turn heat to low and cover. Simmer for 2 hours. Remove bones, slice the clinging meat into shreds, and add meat to soup. If potatoes are still intact, remove from soup and mash; return to soup with the shredded meat.

Makes 6 servings

Split Pea Soup

DAIRY-FREE
EGG-FREE
GLUTEN-FREE

The meat can be cut up and returned to the soup or removed and served with vegetables as a main course. Either way, it will be succulent!

2 cups split green peas
1 pound soup meat (beef)
2 quarts water
1 onion, diced fine
2 whole carrots, scraped

2 sprigs parsley, diced fine
2 celery stalks
1 teaspoon salt
⅛ teaspoon pepper

Rinse and soak split peas for several hours or overnight. Place in a deep pot with soup meat and water. Add remaining ingredients and bring to a boil. Simmer, stirring occasionally, for 2 hours, or until meat is tender. Remove meat, skim soup of any residue, and run rest of ingredients through a sieve or a food mill. Return cut-up meat to soup, if desired.

Makes 8 servings

Black Bean Soup

DAIRY-FREE
EGG-FREE
GLUTEN-FREE

Serve a dish of boiled rice and one of chopped fresh onion to be added to this soup. This can make an important contribution to the menu.

1 pound black kidney beans
3 quarts water
2–3 beef neck bones
1 large onion, diced fine
1 stalk celery, diced fine

1 clove garlic, crushed
1 bay leaf
½ teaspoon salt
¼ teaspoon pepper
Juice of ½ lemon

Soak beans overnight in the water. Add bones, onion, celery, garlic, bay leaf, salt, pepper, and lemon juice. Bring to a boil, then reduce heat and simmer, covered, for 4–5 hours. Soup is ready when most of the beans have softened and disintegrated.

Makes 8–10 servings

Tomato Soup

DAIRY-FREE
EGG-FREE
GLUTEN-FREE

Make your own tomato soup and listen to the raves. Homemade is still the best!

2 meaty beef neck bones
1 28-ounce can tomatoes in natural juice
3 cups water
3 tablespoons rice
1 onion, diced
1 teaspoon sugar
½ teaspoon salt
¼ teaspoon pepper
¼ teaspoon basil

Place neck bones in a heavy saucepan. Add tomatoes, water, rice, and onion. Stir. Add sugar, salt, pepper, and basil. Bring to a boil, reduce heat, cover, and simmer for 2 hours. Stir occasionally. Serve with bits of neck meat.

Makes 6 servings

ENTREES

Beef

Western Hash

DAIRY-FREE
EGG-FREE
GLUTEN-FREE

You won't miss packaged ground beef dinner aids when you know how to season up a potful of your own. Fast and healthful!

2 tablespoons cooking oil
¼ cup finely chopped onion
¼ cup chopped green pepper
1 pound ground beef
½ teaspoon salt
1 teaspoon chili powder
¼ cup pure molasses
¼ cup pure Dijon mustard
2 tablespoons pure Worcestershire sauce
1 16-ounce can tomatoes in natural juice
¼ cup chopped ripe olives
½ teaspoon salt
1 cup uncooked regular rice

Heat oil in a large skillet. Add onion and green pepper and cook until onion is tender but not brown. Add ground beef, the ½ teaspoon salt, and chili powder. Brown the beef, breaking into pieces with a fork. While the beef is browning, mix molasses and mustard. Stir in Worcestershire sauce. Add to the beef mixture with tomatoes, olives, and the remaining ½ teaspoon salt. Gradually add rice. Cover; reduce heat and simmer 25–30 minutes or until rice is tender.

Makes 4 servings

Herbed Hamburgers

DAIRY-FREE
EGG-FREE
GLUTEN-FREE

This is the kind of fast food hamburger that is prepared quicker than you could travel to buy one.

1 pound ground beef	¼ teaspoon pepper
2 tablespoons grated onion	¼ teaspoon marjoram
1 teaspoon pure soy sauce	¼ teaspoon thyme
½ teaspoon salt	

Combine beef, onion, soy sauce, salt, pepper, marjoram, and thyme. Form into 4 hamburgers. Broil about 10 minutes, depending on degree of rareness desired.

Makes 4 servings

Chili Beef on Rice

DAIRY-FREE
EGG-FREE
GLUTEN-FREE

This is for those who love the taste of chili in their beef. Add some more if you have a hankering for it!

1½ pounds ground beef	1 teaspoon chili powder
1 tablespoon cooking oil	⅛ teaspoon pepper
1 cup chopped onions	1 16-ounce can tomatoes
1 cup finely diced green	in natural juices
pepper	3 cups cooked rice
1 teaspoon salt	

Brown beef in oil; then add onions and green pepper. Cook until onions are limp, mixing with a fork. Add salt, chili powder, and pepper. Stir in tomatoes. Cover and simmer about 35 minutes, stirring occasionally to break up the tomatoes. Serve over hot cooked rice.

Makes 6 servings

Meat and Vegetable Chili

DAIRY-FREE
EGG-FREE
GLUTEN-FREE

Here's the kind of meal-in-one that can be cooked while making dinner one night and then refrigerated. Voilà! You'll have dinner all ready for tomorrow.

1 pound ground beef
½ cup chopped onion
1 clove garlic, minced
¼ cup chopped celery
½ cup chopped green pepper
1 bay leaf
1 tablespoon chili powder
1 cup diced pared white turnip

4 cups diced peeled tomatoes
1½ cups beef bouillon
  (may be canned)
1 teaspoon salt
¼ teaspoon dried oregano
¼ teaspoon dried basil
⅛ teaspoon Tabasco sauce
1 tablespoon brown sugar

In a Dutch oven, cook beef over medium heat until browned and separated into bits. Add onion, garlic, celery, and green pepper. Cook until vegetables are tender, about 10 minutes. Add bay leaf, chili powder, turnip, tomatoes, bouillon, salt, oregano, basil, Tabasco, and sugar. Cook, uncovered, over low heat for 1 hour, stirring occasionally.

Makes 4 servings

Stuffed Peppers

DAIRY-FREE
EGG-FREE
GLUTEN-FREE

This is a great use for extra peppers from your garden or your local market. The raisins add a sweet tang.

6 green peppers
2 cups boiling water
1 pound ground beef
1 small onion, grated
1 clove garlic, minced

½ teaspoon salt
¼ teaspoon pepper
1½ cups tomato juice
½ cup seedless raisins

Cut green peppers in half lengthwise and remove seeds, stems, and pith. Cook in boiling water for 5 minutes, until tender but still firm. Drain and arrange in a baking pan cut sides up. Combine beef, onion, garlic, salt, pepper, ½ cup of the tomato juice, and seedless raisins. Fill each pepper with this mixture. Pour remaining 1 cup tomato juice around the peppers. Cover the baking pan with a lid or with aluminum foil. Bake in a 350° F. oven for 45 minutes, then remove cover and bake 15 minutes more.

Makes 6 servings

Beef Stew

DAIRY-FREE
EGG-FREE
GLUTEN-FREE

Don't omit the bay leaves from this recipe. They give just the punch of flavor that can make a stew sublime!

2 pounds boned beef cubes
1 6-ounce can tomato sauce
½ cup water
½ teaspoon salt
½ teaspoon garlic powder
½ teaspoon thyme
2 bay leaves
2 onions, sliced thin
6 carrots, scraped and cut into chunks
6 stalks celery, cut into chunks
6 potatoes, peeled and cut into chunks

Place beef cubes in the bottom of a heavy saucepan. Pour combined tomato sauce and water over the beef. Add salt, garlic powder, thyme, and bay leaves. Add onions, carrots, celery, and potatoes. Mix well. Cover and bake in a 325° F. oven or simmer on top of the range for 1½–2 hours.

Makes 6 servings

Pepper Steak

DAIRY-FREE
EGG-FREE
GLUTEN-FREE

If your wok is gathering dust in the pantry, this is a good recipe to try in it. Have all ingredients ready before you start to cook, and you'll be done before you know it!

1½ pounds beef steak
¼ cup salad oil
1 large onion, sliced thin
4 green peppers, seeded and cut up
1 clove garlic, minced
½ teaspoon salt
¼ teaspoon pepper
¼ teaspoon ground ginger
1 cup unsweetened pineapple juice
1 tablespoon pure soy sauce
1 tablespoon cornstarch

Cut steak diagonally across the grain into thin strips and then cut the strips into 2-inch pieces. Heat the oil in a skillet or a wok; add the meat and quickly brown it on all sides. Add onion, peppers, garlic, salt, pepper, and ginger. Cook over medium heat, stirring constantly for several minutes, until peppers are tender. Combine pineapple juice, soy sauce, and cornstarch, mixing until smooth; stir into the meat mixture and bring to a boil. Stir constantly while mixture bubbles and then clears. Serve over cooked rice, if desired.

Makes 6 servings

Beef Shashlik

DAIRY-FREE
EGG-FREE
GLUTEN-FREE

The secret to this recipe is to marinate it for a long time and mix often. An easy way is to put all into a plastic bag and then into the bowl. Fasten the bag and flip it every so often.

2 pounds boneless sirloin steak
1 cup salad oil
1 onion, grated fine
2 teaspoons dried oregano
1 bay leaf
½ teaspoon salt
12 small white onions, parboiled
2 green peppers, cut into 2-inch squares
2 large tomatoes, cut into sixths
12 large fresh mushroom caps

Trim fat from meat and cut into 2-inch cubes. Combine oil, grated onion, oregano, and bay leaf in a deep bowl; add meat and mix well. Cover bowl tightly and refrigerate for at least 8 hours, mixing meat in the marinade every few hours. When ready to cook, remove meat from marinade. Sprinkle with salt. Place alternately on 6 long skewers with onions, pepper chunks, tomatoes, and mushrooms. Brush all lightly with the remaining marinade. Place on a broiler pan and broil for about 8 minutes for rare meat, turning once and brushing again with marinade.

Makes 6 servings

Stuffed Flank Steak

DAIRY-FREE
EGG-FREE
GLUTEN-FREE

This is a wonderful way to stretch that flank steak to serve six. And what a fruitful stuffing!

1 flank steak (1½–2 pounds)
Salt and pepper
¼ cup finely chopped onion
2 apples, peeled, cored,
  and sliced
8 pitted prunes
2 tablespoons corn oil

1 cup water
1½ cups apple juice
2 tablespoons cornstarch
1 teaspoon salt
1 tablespoon brown sugar
¼ teaspoon onion powder

Trim excess fat and membrane from steak. Score both sides and sprinkle with salt and pepper. Pound both sides with a meat mallet. Sprinkle one side with onion; arrange apples and prunes in the center across the short side of the steak. Fold in thirds and tie securely. In a Dutch oven or a large skillet, heat corn oil over medium heat. Add steak; brown on all sides. Reduce heat; add water. Cover and simmer 1 hour or until meat is fork-tender. Remove meat; keep warm. Gradually stir apple juice into cornstarch until smooth. Stir into pan juices. Stir in 1 teaspoon salt, brown sugar, and onion powder. Cook over medium heat, stirring constantly until mixture thickens and comes to a boil. Serve gravy over meat.

Makes 6 servings

Flank Steak Teriyaki

DAIRY-FREE
EGG-FREE
GLUTEN-FREE

The best of both worlds—an Oriental flavor with an All-American steak

1 flank steak (about 2 pounds)   ½ teaspoon ginger
¼ cup pure soy sauce   1 clove crushed garlic
1 tablespoon brown sugar   1 tablespoon salad oil

Place flank steak on a broiling rack. Combine remaining ingredients and brush half the mixture on top of the steak. Broil 10 minutes. Turn and brush remaining sauce on top of steak. Broil 5–10 minutes more, depending on desired degree of rareness. Slice steak on an extreme diagonal across the grain, in thin slices.

Makes 4 servings

Beef Brisket Pot Roast

DAIRY-FREE
EGG-FREE
GLUTEN-FREE

Purchase the first cut of fresh brisket of beef—the second cut is already too fatty. Then cook it slowly on low heat for the tenderest and tastiest meat!

4–5 pounds beef brisket
2 onions, sliced thin
1 teaspoon salt
¼ teaspoon pepper
2 bay leaves
1 cup water
1 teaspoon paprika

Place brisket in a Dutch oven. Spread onions around meat. Sprinkle with salt and pepper. Place bay leaves in pot. Add water around sides. Sprinkle with paprika. Cover and roast in a 300° F. oven for 3–3½ hours, or until fork-tender. Serve in thick slices with pan gravy.

Makes 8 servings

Baked Brisket

DAIRY-FREE
EGG-FREE
GLUTEN-FREE

Here's another brisket, but with vegetables added to make it a meal in one pot.

About 4 pounds beef brisket
½ teaspoon salt
¼ teaspoon pepper
½ teaspoon paprika
2 onions, sliced thin
2 cups water
2 bay leaves
4 carrots, scraped and sliced thin
4 potatoes, peeled and quartered
Optional: 2 turnips, peeled and quartered
          1½ cups fresh green beans, trimmed

Place brisket in a Dutch oven. Season with salt, pepper, and paprika. Cover with sliced onions. Pour water around the brisket. Add bay leaves and sliced carrots. Cover and bake in a 325° F. oven for 2 hours. Add potatoes (and turnips, if desired) and continue baking, covered, for an additional 30 minutes—adding green beans, if desired, after 15 minutes—or until brisket and potatoes are tender. Remove bay leaves. Slice brisket and serve with potatoes and gravy.

Makes 8–10 servings

Pot Roast

DAIRY-FREE
EGG-FREE
GLUTEN-FREE

Beef chuck is a good cut for this recipe, or you can use any other cut that is suitable for long, low-heat cookery.

¼ cup corn oil
1 boneless beef pot roast (4–5 pounds)
2 cups chopped onion
2½ cups beef stock or water
2 teaspoons salt
1 teaspoon pepper
2 crushed bay leaves
8 small potatoes, peeled
1 pound whole green beans
⅓ cup cornstarch
⅓ cup water

In a Dutch oven or a large kettle, heat corn oil over medium heat. Add meat. Brown on all sides. Stir in onion, beef stock, salt, pepper, and bay leaves. Cover. Bake in a 350° F. oven for about 2½ hours, or until meat is almost tender. Add potatoes. Cover and cook ½ hour, or until meat and potatoes are tender. Add green beans. Cover and cook an additional 10–15 minutes, or until beans are crisp-tender. Transfer meat and vegetables to platter. Stir together cornstarch and water until smooth. Add to liquid in Dutch oven. Bring to a boil over medium heat, stirring constantly, and boil 1 minute. Serve gravy over meat and vegetables.

Makes about 8 servings

Veal

Veal Pot Roast

DAIRY-FREE
EGG-FREE
GLUTEN-FREE

Leftovers of this roast are delicious cold for the next day's lunch. Don't omit the garlic—it gives depth of flavor to the otherwise delicate meat.

1 boned and tied veal shoulder roast (about 3 pounds)
1 clove garlic, halved lengthwise
1 tablespoon paprika
1 teaspoon salt
¼ teaspoon pepper
3 tablespoons cooking oil
1 onion, diced
1 cup water
Sprig of fresh dillweed
4 carrots, scraped and cut into 2-inch chunks

Rub the veal roast with the cut sides of garlic; reserve garlic. Combine paprika, salt, and pepper; rub all over the surface of the roast. Heat oil in a deep kettle or Dutch oven; sauté the onion until lightly golden. Add reserved garlic to oil. Add veal and brown on all sides. Remove garlic. Add water, dill, and carrots. Cover and simmer 1½ hours (about 30 minutes to the pound).

Makes 6–8 servings

Breast of Veal with Rice Stuffing

DAIRY-FREE
EGG-FREE
GLUTEN-FREE

Trim this meat cut of all excess fat. The stuffing helps the meat stretch and provides a built-in side dish.

1 breast of veal (about 4 pounds)   ½ teaspoon salt
2 cups cooked rice   ⅛ teaspoon pepper
2 tablespoons minced parsley   ½ teaspoon paprika
1 teaspoon grated lemon rind   ¼ teaspoon garlic salt
½ teaspoon basil

Have butcher slit a pocket into the breast of veal for stuffing. Combine cooked rice, parsley, lemon rind, basil, salt, and pepper. Stuff into veal pocket. Place breast of veal in a roasting pan; sprinkle surface with paprika and garlic salt. Roast in a 350° F. oven for 2–2½ hours, or until browned and tender.

Makes 6 servings

Lamb

Irish Stew

DAIRY-FREE
EGG-FREE
GLUTEN-FREE

Simple and hearty stew is a favorite of most everyone. Serve with a crisp green salad and stewed fruit for dessert.

2 pounds cubed lamb
2 large onions, sliced
2 tablespoons cooking oil
2 tablespoons minced parsley
1 teaspoon salt
¼ teaspoon pepper
1½ cups water
4 large potatoes, cut into chunks
4 carrots, scraped and cut into chunks
2 stalks celery, cut into chunks

Brown lamb cubes and onions in oil in a large heavy saucepan. Add parsley, salt, and pepper. Add water. Cover and simmer for 1 hour, until tender. Add potatoes, carrots, and celery; cover and simmer for ½ hour longer, or until tender.

Makes 4 servings

Lamb Chops Italienne

DAIRY-FREE
EGG-FREE
GLUTEN-FREE

Why have plain, dull broiled lamb chops when you can spark the flavor with herbs and more? Here's a savory way to do it!

6 large shoulder lamb chops (about 2 pounds)
¼ cup white vinegar
2 tablespoons lemon juice
1 tablespoon olive oil
1 clove garlic, crushed
¾ teaspoon oregano
½ teaspoon salt
¼ teaspoon pepper

Arrange lamb chops on a rack in a broiling pan. Combine vinegar, lemon juice, olive oil, garlic, oregano, salt, and pepper. Brush mixture on chops and broil for about 8 minutes. Turn chops, brush the remaining mixture on the other side, and broil 8 minutes more, or until done to your taste.

Makes 4–6 servings

Apricot-Glazed Lamb Chops

DAIRY-FREE
EGG-FREE
GLUTEN-FREE

Here's a way to perk up your chops. A lovely combination of apricot and rosemary.

6 large shoulder lamb chops
½ cup canned unsweetened apricot nectar
½ teaspoon rosemary
¼ teaspoon ginger

Arrange the lamb chops on a broiling rack. Combine apricot nectar with rosemary and ginger; spoon half of the mixture over the chops. Broil for 4 minutes. Turn the chops and spoon the remaining mixture over them. Broil for 4 minutes longer, or until desired doneness is achieved.

Makes 6 servings

Roast Leg of Lamb

DAIRY-FREE
EGG-FREE
GLUTEN-FREE

It's so easy to prepare this roast. Just season and then let the oven do the rest!

1 leg of lamb roast (about 5 pounds)
1 clove garlic, minced
1 teaspoon salt
¼ teaspoon pepper
½ teaspoon paprika
½ teaspoon rosemary
1 onion, finely diced
2 tablespoons white vinegar
¼ cup olive oil

Rub lamb with a mixture of garlic, salt, pepper, paprika, and rosemary. Place on a rack in a roasting pan. Combine onion, vinegar, and oil; pour over lamb. Place in a preheated 350° F. oven and roast for about 20 minutes to the pound for rare, 25 minutes for medium, 30 minutes for well done. Let roast stand for 15 minutes—it will carve more easily.

Makes 6–8 servings

Pork

Pork Chop Casserole

DAIRY-FREE
EGG-FREE
GLUTEN-FREE

Pork chops and dried fruit go so well together. Here they are enhanced with apple as well.

8 loin pork chops, ½ inch thick
½ teaspoon salt
⅛ teaspoon pepper
4 tablespoons dairy-free margarine
1 finely diced onion
1⅓ cups enriched precooked rice
1⅓ cups water
1 cup peeled and diced tart apples
1 cup chopped prunes
¼ teaspoon poultry seasoning
¼ teaspoon sage

Trim excess fat from pork chops; sprinkle with salt and pepper. Brown chops quickly in 2 tablespoons margarine in a large skillet; drain on paper towels. Pour drippings from skillet; melt remaining 2 tablespoons margarine in skillet and sauté onion. Combine rice, water, apples, prunes, poultry seasoning, and sage in a casserole greased with margarine. Add sautéed onion and mix well. Arrange pork chops on top of rice mixture. Cover tightly and bake in a 350°F. oven for 45 minutes, or until chops are tender and well done.

Makes 4 servings

Pineapple Pepper Pork Chops

DAIRY-FREE
EGG-FREE
GLUTEN-FREE

Cook pork chops until there is no trace of pink in the juices or meat. The seasonings in this recipe blend into a flavorful offering.

2 tablespoons corn oil
4 pork chops, 1 inch thick
1 8-ounce can sliced pineapple or pineapple chunks with
    juice
1 tablespoon pure soy sauce
¼ teaspoon dried thyme leaves
½ teaspoon salt
¼ teaspoon pepper
2 tablespoons cornstarch
½ cup beef stock or Chicken Broth (see recipe)
¼ cup chopped green pepper
4 green pepper rings

In skillet heat corn oil over medium heat. Add pork chops. Brown on all sides. Place chops in a shallow baking dish. Mix together pineapple juice, soy sauce, thyme, salt, and pepper. Stir together cornstarch and stock until smooth. Stir into pineapple mixture. Pour over pork chops. Add chopped green pepper. Cover. Bake in a 350° F. oven 45 minutes or until pork chops are tender. Remove from oven. Top pork chops with pineapple and green pepper. Continue baking, uncovered, 5 minutes, or until pineapple is heated through and gravy thickened.

Makes 4 servings

Honey-Citrus Pork Chops

DAIRY-FREE
EGG-FREE
GLUTEN-FREE

Here's a great way to make pork chops with a sweet and tangy sauce.

4 pork chops, 1-inch thick
¼ cup orange juice
2 tablespoons lemon juice
2 tablespoons honey
½ teaspoon dry mustard
⅛ teaspoon pepper
⅛ teaspoon allspice
½ teaspoon ginger
⅛ teaspoon nutmeg

Place pork chops in a flat baking dish. Combine orange juice, lemon juice, honey, dry mustard, pepper, allspice, ginger, and nutmeg; mix well. Pour the sauce over the pork chops and marinate for several hours, turning once or twice. Place chops and sauce in the broiler, about 6 inches from heat and broil, basting frequently with sauce. Cook for 15 minutes on each side or until well done.

Makes 4 servings

Poultry

Roast Chicken

DAIRY-FREE
EGG-FREE
GLUTEN-FREE

When the doctor instructs you to cook food in the simplest manner, here's a delicious way to prepare chicken with just a few ingredients.

1 roasting chicken
  (about 5 pounds)
1 lemon
1 teaspoon salt

½ teaspoon paprika
2 sprigs parsley
1 small onion, sliced
1 cup water

Clean and wash chicken thoroughly; arrange in an open pan. Cut lemon in half and squeeze the juice over the surfaces of the chicken, including the interior. Sprinkle salt both inside and out. Sprinkle the skin with paprika. Tuck remaining squeezed-out lemon halves and parsley into the chicken. Place onion slices around the base of the chicken and pour water into the pan. Roast in a 350° F. oven about 2 hours, basting occasionally with pan juices. Remove lemon rinds and parsley from chicken cavity before serving.

Makes 4–6 servings

Chicken Italienne

DAIRY-FREE
EGG-FREE
GLUTEN-FREE

If you can substitute fresh mushrooms, this will taste so much better. Brown rice has more nutrients than the refined white variety.

3 pounds chicken pieces
¼ teaspoon salt
⅛ teaspoon ground black pepper
1 teaspoon garlic powder
3 tablespoons vegetable oil
1 4-ounce can sliced mushrooms with liquid
½ cup dry white wine
¾ teaspoon rosemary
3 cups hot cooked brown rice

Sprinkle chicken pieces with salt, pepper, and garlic powder; sauté in hot vegetable oil. Pour off fat. Add mushrooms, wine, and rosemary leaves. Cover and simmer 45–55 minutes, or until chicken is tender. Serve over hot cooked rice.

Makes 6 servings

Chicken à l' Orange

DAIRY-FREE
EGG-FREE
GLUTEN-FREE

This sounds almost too simple to be delicious. But try it and your taste buds will say, "Hooray!"

2 broiler chickens
  (about 3 pounds each)
½ teaspoon salt

2 cups orange juice
½ teaspoon onion salt
½ teaspoon paprika

Arrange chickens in a roasting pan. Salt cavities. Pour orange juice generously over the chickens, spooning it into the cavities as well. Sprinkle chickens with onion salt and paprika. Place in a 350° F. oven and roast for 1 hour, occasionally basting with pan juices. When done, remove chickens from pan and pour ½ cup boiling water into pan to make gravy from the scrapings. Pour gravy over chicken and serve.

Makes 8 servings

Chicken Fricassee II

DAIRY-FREE
EGG-FREE
GLUTEN-FREE

Here's a gluten-free way to serve a thick-gravied fricassee. Substitute 2 cups of milk for the broth when making the creamy gravy for someone without a dairy allergy.

1 broiler chicken, cut up
2 carrots, quartered
1 stalk celery, halved
1 medium onion
2 sprigs parsley
1½ teaspoons salt

¾ teaspoon dried thyme leaves
⅛ teaspoon white pepper
5 cups water
⅓ cup cornstarch
Chopped parsley (optional)

In a large kettle, place the chicken, carrots, celery, onion, parsley, salt, thyme, and pepper. Add water. Bring to a boil, reduce heat, cover, and simmer 45 minutes, or until the chicken is fork-tender. Strain broth, discarding vegetables. Return 4 cups of broth to the kettle. Stir together cornstarch and remaining broth until smooth. Stir into broth in kettle. Bring to boil over medium heat, stirring constantly, and boil 1 minute. Add chicken and heat. Serve over rice in soup bowls. If desired, sprinkle with chopped parsley.

Makes 4 servings

Chili Chicken

DAIRY-FREE
EGG-FREE
GLUTEN-FREE

In case you thought that chilied food only referred to beef combinations, here's the way to pep up some leftover chicken. Whenever possible, use brown rice.

1 cup chopped onion
½ cup chopped green pepper
1 clove garlic, crushed
1 tablespoon dairy-free margarine
2 cups Chicken Broth (see recipe)
1 6-ounce can tomato paste
2 tablespoons chopped parsley
1 teaspoon chili powder
½ teaspoon salt
¼ teaspoon pepper
¼ teaspoon oregano
2 cups chopped cooked chicken
3 cups hot cooked brown rice

Cook onion, green pepper, and garlic in margarine until onion is soft but not brown. Stir in chicken broth, tomato paste, parsley, chili powder, salt, pepper, and oregano. Cover and simmer about 10 minutes. Add chicken and cook 5 minutes longer. Serve over hot cooked rice.

Makes 6 servings

Chicken Stew

DAIRY-FREE
EGG-FREE
GLUTEN-FREE

Don't forget the sprigs of fresh dillweed. They make chicken taste very special.

2 broiler chickens (about 3 pounds each)
1 onion, sliced
2 sweet green peppers, cut into cubes
½ pound mushrooms, sliced
4 carrots, scraped and cut into chunks
4 celery stalks, cut into chunks
4 potatoes, peeled and quartered
2 sprigs fresh dillweed
2 sprigs fresh parsley
1 cup water
¼ cup lemon juice
1 teaspoon salt
¼ teaspoon pepper

Wash, dry, and arrange chickens in a Dutch oven with a tight-fitting lid. Add onion, peppers, mushrooms, carrots, celery, potatoes, dillweed, and parsley around the chickens. Pour in water and lemon juice. Sprinkle salt and pepper over all. Cover and place in a 350° F. oven for 1½ hours.

Makes 8 servings

Chicken and Cashews

DAIRY-FREE
EGG-FREE
GLUTEN-FREE

The cashews make this elegant enough for company dinner. If you can't find red pepper in the market, double up on the green variety.

2 tablespoons pure soy sauce
2 tablespoons water
2 teaspoons cornstarch
¼ teaspoon white pepper
2 whole chicken breasts, skinned, boned, and diced (1½ cups)
3 tablespoons corn oil
3 ounces whole mushrooms, sliced
½ cup diced green pepper
½ cup diced red pepper
1 tablespoon cornstarch
½ cup Chicken Broth (see recipe)
2 cups cooked rice
¾ cup salted cashews

Stir together soy sauce, water, 2 teaspoons cornstarch, and white pepper until smooth. Mix in chicken. Marinate ½ hour at room temperature. In a wok or a 4-quart saucepan, heat corn oil over medium-high heat. Add mushrooms and green and red peppers. Cook over high heat, stirring constantly, for 1 minute. Remove and set aside. Add chicken. Cook over high heat, stirring constantly, for 2 minutes, or until tender. Stir together 1 tablespoon cornstarch and chicken broth. Add to the wok. Bring to a boil over medium heat, stirring constantly, and boil 1 minute. Stir in vegetables. Cook until heated through. Spoon over a bed of hot cooked rice. Top with cashews.

Makes 4 servings

Chicken Paprikash

DAIRY-FREE
EGG-FREE
GLUTEN-FREE

If you can find imported sweet Hungarian paprika, use it and increase the amount if desired. Makes a memorable chicken dinner.

2 frying chickens (about
 3 pounds each), cut up
1 teaspoon salt
1 tablespoon paprika
2 tablespoons salad oil

1 onion, sliced thin
1 cup Chicken Broth
 (see recipe)
1 tablespoon cornstarch
¼ cup water

Wash and pat dry the chicken parts. Sprinkle with salt and sprinkle heavily with paprika. Heat oil in a Dutch oven; sauté the onion until transparent. Add chicken and brown lightly, turning constantly. Add broth. Cover and simmer for 1 hour, or until chicken parts are tender. Stir cornstarch into water; add several tablespoons of the hot gravy. Then stir into the gravy and continue to stir and cook until gravy is thickened.

Makes 8 servings

Skillet Barbecued Chicken

DAIRY-FREE
EGG-FREE
GLUTEN-FREE

It's so easy to get this dinner together. Cook it tonight while you eat another meal, then refrigerate and have it all ready to heat for tomorrow's dinner. A cook-and-coast way to lead a busy life!

1 fryer chicken (about
 3 pounds), cut up
2 tablespoons olive oil
1 onion, diced
1 15-ounce can tomato sauce
1 tablespoon white vinegar

1 tablespoon brown sugar
1 teaspoon pure
 Worcestershire sauce
½ teaspoon salt
¼ teaspoon pepper

Brown chicken parts in olive oil, push aside, and add onion to cook until golden. Combine tomato sauce, vinegar, brown sugar, Worcestershire sauce, salt, and pepper. Pour over chicken. Cover skillet and turn heat low. Simmer for 30 minutes, or until tender. Add water to pan if needed.

Makes 4 servings

Chicken Grandmère

DAIRY-FREE
EGG-FREE
GLUTEN-FREE

Here's the old-fashioned way to cook a flavorful chicken in the pot.

2 fryer chickens (about 3 pounds each), cut up
6 cups water
2 cups sliced celery stalks and leaves
¾ cup parsley sprigs
2 medium onions, sliced
2 teaspoons salt
1 bay leaf
¼ teaspoon thyme leaves
6 tablespoons cornstarch
Cooked rice

Place the chicken in a 6-quart kettle; cover with water. Add celery, parsley, onions, salt, bay leaf, and thyme. Cover, bring to a boil, reduce heat, and simmer 1¼ hours, or until chicken is tender. Remove chicken and discard bones. Strain broth; measure 6 cups, adding boiling water if necessary. Return 5 cups of broth to the kettle; mix together remaining broth and cornstarch until smooth. Stir the broth into the kettle. Bring to a boil, stirring constantly, and boil 1 minute, until the mixture is slightly thickened. Add chicken and heat. Serve over rice in soup bowls.

Makes 8 servings

Oriental Broiled Chicken

DAIRY-FREE
EGG-FREE
GLUTEN-FREE

If you have a hankering for a sweet coating on your broiled chicken, this will be most satisfying. By the time you make a salad and steam a vegetable or two, this will be ready.

1 cup orange juice
¼ cup honey
¼ cup soy sauce
1 clove garlic, crushed
½ teaspoon powdered ginger
2 broiler chickens (about 3 pounds each), quartered

Combine orange juice, honey, soy sauce, garlic, and ginger, stirring well until honey is dissolved. Arrange chicken quarters in a broiling pan. Pour half of the orange juice mixture over the chicken. Broil for 15 minutes. Turn chicken quarters and pour the remaining orange mixture over all. Broil for an additional 15 minutes, or until chicken is tender.

Makes 8 servings

Hawaiian Chicken

DAIRY-FREE
EGG-FREE
GLUTEN-FREE

Pineapple has a way of dressing up a simple meal. Here it is a marinade, and it adorns the finished dish. That's getting kitchen mileage!

2 broiler chickens (about 3 pounds each), cut up
1 16-ounce can pineapple chunks with juice
¼ cup pure soy sauce
½ teaspoon ground ginger
½ teaspoon garlic powder
1 teaspoon cornstarch

Place chicken parts in a deep bowl. Combine pineapple chunks with juice, soy sauce, ginger, and garlic powder; pour over chicken and refrigerate, covered, for several hours. When ready to cook, remove chicken from marinade and place in a flat baking dish. Add cornstarch to marinade and mix until smooth; then pour into a saucepan and cook, stirring constantly, until mixture thickens. Pour mixture over chicken. Place in a 350° F. oven for 1½ hours, spooning sauce over chicken several times during the baking.

Makes 8 servings

Chicken Stew II

DAIRY-FREE
EGG-FREE
GLUTEN-FREE

When is a soup not a soup? When it's a stew with plenty of gravy to spoon up. Here's a lovely supper dish that's easy on the palate.

2 chicken fryers (about 3 pounds each), cut up
2 teaspoons salt
1 bay leaf
¼ teaspoon thyme leaves
5 cups water
2 cups celery, cut into 3-inch strips
2 cups carrots, cut into 3-inch strips
12 small white onions
⅓ cup cornstarch
1 cup water

Place chicken pieces, salt, bay leaf, thyme, and water in a large kettle. Bring to a boil, reduce heat, and simmer, covered, for 30 minutes. Add celery, carrots, and onions; simmer, covered, for about 10 minutes, or until vegetables are tender. Mix cornstarch and 1 cup water; stir into chicken mixture. Bring to a boil, stirring constantly, and boil 1 minute. Serve in soup plates.

Makes 8 servings

Brunswick Stew

DAIRY-FREE
EGG-FREE
GLUTEN-FREE

In the southern part of the country this stew has as many versions as there are cooks. The following recipe leans toward the Virginia version.

1 chicken (about 3 pounds), cut up
1½ cups water
1 onion, sliced thin
1 16-ounce can tomatoes in natural juice
1 teaspoon salt
¼ teaspoon pepper
2 potatoes, peeled and cut into chunks
1 12-ounce can whole corn niblets, drained
1 8-ounce can okra, drained
1 teaspoon pure Worcestershire sauce

Place chicken parts in a deep saucepan. Add water, onion, tomatoes, salt, and pepper. Simmer, covered, for 15 minutes. Add potatoes, corn, okra, and Worcestershire sauce. Simmer, covered, for 30 minutes more, or until chicken is tender.

Makes 4 servings

Roast Duckling

DAIRY-FREE
EGG-FREE
GLUTEN-FREE

The secret of duck cookery is to turn the heat high at the end, pierce the skin, and let all the fat melt away. The fat is needed to keep the duck afloat, when it's alive. We humans are much better off without it.

1 duckling (about 5 pounds)   1 teaspoon salt
1 orange   ¼ teaspoon garlic salt

Arrange duck on a rack in an open roasting pan. Cut orange in half; squeeze generously over skin of duck and then tuck the remaining orange rind into the cavity of the duck. Sprinkle skin of duck with salt and garlic salt. Roast in a 300° F. oven for 2 hours, and then turn heat up to 500° F. for 15 minutes. Pierce the skin of the duck all over with a fork as it roasts, to permit the layer of fat under the skin to run off. The high heat at the end of the roasting will ensure the melting of any remaining fat and the final crisping of the duck.

Makes 4 servings

Chicken Livers and Mushrooms

DAIRY-FREE
EGG-FREE
GLUTEN-FREE

Serve these poached livers on rice or mashed potatoes. Add some tomato sauce for a perfect sauce for pasta (if pasta is allowed). Liver is high in iron and essential nutrients.

½ cup Chicken Broth (see recipe)
2 onions, sliced thin
1½ pounds chicken livers
½ pound fresh mushrooms, sliced
2 tablespoons minced parsley
1 teaspoon paprika
½ teaspoon salt
⅛ teaspoon pepper

Pour chicken broth into a large skillet. Heat and add sliced onions; cook until translucent. Add chicken livers and mushrooms; sprinkle with parsley, paprika, salt, and pepper. Cover and simmer for 10 minutes, or until livers are tender.

Makes 4 servings

Fish

Baked Haddock

DAIRY-FREE
EGG-FREE
GLUTEN-FREE

If you dislike bland-tasting fish, here's the way to sauce it up. Be sure to test the fish with a fork to see whether it is done (if it flakes easily, it's ready), then serve at once. Nothing is worse than overcooked fish!

2 pounds haddock fillets
1 8-ounce can tomato sauce
1 small onion, diced
1 clove garlic, minced
½ green pepper, diced fine
2 tablespoons lemon juice
½ teaspoon salt
⅛ teaspoon pepper

Arrange haddock fillets in a greased baking dish. Combine remaining ingredients in a small saucepan; simmer for 5 minutes. Pour sauce over fish. Bake in a 350° F. oven for 20 minutes, or until fish flakes easily.

Makes 6 servings

Baked Bass

DAIRY-FREE
EGG-FREE
GLUTEN-FREE

Here's an easy way to cook a whole fish. If desired, place strips of bacon over the fish before baking.

1 cleaned whole bass
  (3–4 pounds)
¼ cup lemon juice
½ teaspoon salt
¼ teaspoon pepper
2 cups tomato juice
1 small onion, chopped
1 stalk celery chopped

Place bass in a roasting pan. Pour lemon juice over one side, and turn the bass so that the lemon juice coats the other side. Sprinkle with salt and pepper. Pour tomato juice around the fish. Add chopped onion and celery. Place in a preheated 350° F. oven and bake for 30–40 minutes, or until fish flakes easily when tested with a fork. Place on a large hot platter and pour pan juices over fish.

Makes 4 servings

Boiled Salmon

DAIRY-FREE
EGG-FREE
GLUTEN-FREE

Don't forget the vinegar in the boiling water. It is just the trick to keep the fish flesh firm.

4 small salmon steaks (about 2 pounds)
Boiling water
1 lemon, sliced thin
1 sprig fresh dillweed
1 sprig fresh parsley
1 teaspoon vinegar
½ teaspoon salt

Place salmon steaks on a rack in the bottom of a fish poacher or large skillet. Cover with boiling water. Add sliced lemon, dillweed, parsley, vinegar, and salt. Simmer for about 10 minutes, or until fish flakes easily but holds its shape. Remove fish carefully and serve hot or chilled.

Makes 4 servings

Shrimp in Parsley Sauce

DAIRY-FREE
EGG-FREE
GLUTEN-FREE

Here's a gourmet way to prepare shrimp. Leave about 20 minutes to peel and devein the little rascals–it's time-consuming but worth it.

1 tablespoon olive oil
1 clove garlic, minced
1 scallion, sliced fine
¼ cup finely chopped fresh parsley
1 pound shrimp, peeled and deveined
1 cup Chicken Broth (see recipe)
1 tablespoon lemon juice
2 teaspoons cornstarch
¼ teaspoon salt
⅛ teaspoon pepper

Heat olive oil in a skillet; add garlic and scallion and sauté for several minutes. Add parsley and shrimp; cook and stir for a minute. Then add combined mixture of chicken broth, lemon juice, cornstarch, salt, and pepper. Cover and cook for 3 minutes. Remove cover; stir and cook until mixture thickens. Serve over rice, if desired.

Makes 4 servings

Shrimp Oriental

DAIRY-FREE
EGG-FREE
GLUTEN-FREE

If you can get fresh ginger root, grate a bit into this as you sauté the shrimp. Include the green tops of the scallions for color and subtle flavor.

1½ teaspoons cornstarch
½ teaspoon salt
⅛ teaspoon ginger
1 tablespoon lemon juice

1 pound shrimp, shelled
  and deveined
2 tablespoons corn oil
1 scallion, chopped

Combine cornstarch, salt, and ginger. Stir in lemon juice. Toss with shrimp, coating evenly. Heat corn oil in a skillet. Add shrimp and sauté over medium heat 5–7 minutes, stirring occasionally. Add scallions.

Makes 4 servings

Broiled Scampi

DAIRY-FREE
EGG-FREE
GLUTEN-FREE

Marinate the shrimp in the oil mixture for several hours in the refrigerator—it will taste ever so much better. It's a fast cooker, so don't let it burn!

1 pound large shrimp, peeled and cleaned, with tails left on
2 tablespoons olive oil
1 clove garlic, crushed
1 tablespoon minced fresh parsley
½ teaspoon brown sugar
½ teaspoon salt
¼ teaspoon pepper
Lemon wedges

Split the shrimp into a butterfly shape by slitting down the back and pressing flat, leaving the tail intact. Combine oil, garlic, parsley, brown sugar, salt, and pepper. Arrange shrimp on a broiling pan, brush with oil mixture, and broil for 3 minutes on each side. Serve with lemon wedges.

Makes 4 servings

Citrus-Marinated Shrimp

DAIRY-FREE
EGG-FREE
GLUTEN-FREE

When you need an elegant hors d'oeuvre for a large cocktail party and don't need to look at the price, double this recipe and watch your happy guests scoop them up.

1 pound shrimp
½ lemon, sliced
½ onion, sliced thin
1 sprig parsley
1 bay leaf
Water
1 cup orange juice
½ cup lemon juice
3 tablespoons chopped onion
3 tablespoons chopped green pepper
1 tablespoon chopped parsley
¼ cup salad oil
1 clove crushed garlic
½ teaspoon salt
¼ teaspoon pepper

Wash shrimp, removing shells and cleaning well. Place shrimp in a saucepan with sliced lemon, sliced onion, sprig of parsley, and bay leaf; add water to cover. Cook for about 3 minutes. Drain. Place in a bowl with remaining ingredients and marinate for at least 3 hours before serving. Drain and serve as an hors d'oeuvre or as a first course.

Makes 4 servings

VEGETABLES

Artichokes

DAIRY-FREE
EGG-FREE
GLUTEN-FREE

Here's an easy way to cook an artichoke. Remember to remove the choke during eating or you'll have a fibrous mouthful along the way.

4 whole fresh artichokes
¼ cup lemon juice
¼ cup olive oil
1 clove garlic
2 bay leaves

Cut bottom stems from artichokes so they will stand up evenly. With kitchen scissors, cut sharp points off each leaf. Use a sharp knife to cut the top inch of the artichoke off, and then rap it hard on the cutting board while holding it upside down, to open the leaves a bit. Pour lemon juice into a skillet and roll each artichoke around in the juice to prevent the cut edges from discoloring. Then stand the artichokes up. Drizzle each with olive oil, allowing the excess to flow into the lemon juice in the skillet. Add garlic and bay leaves to the skillet. Fill with ½ inch of water. Cover tightly and simmer for 25 minutes. Test for doneness by pulling at a bottom leaf—if it comes out easily, the artichokes are done. Serve warm.

Makes 4 servings

Asparagus-Banana Salad

DAIRY-FREE
EGG-FREE
GLUTEN-FREE

Why do all salads have to be mixed greens? Here's a way to break that pattern.

1 pound asparagus, cooked and drained	2 tablespoons chopped chives
2 tomatoes, cut into small wedges	2 sprigs chopped parsley
⅓ cup cider vinegar	1 teaspoon salt
½ cup salad oil	1 teaspoon sugar
2 teaspoons lemon juice	½ teaspoon dry mustard
	3 bananas
	Salad greens

Place asparagus in a flat container; add tomatoes. Combine vinegar, oil, lemon juice, chives, parsley, salt, sugar, and dry mustard; pour over asparagus. Cover and refrigerate for several hours. When ready to serve, peel bananas and slice. Add to asparagus and tomatoes; serve on a bed of salad greens.

Makes 4–6 servings

Zesty Green Beans

DAIRY-FREE
EGG-FREE
GLUTEN-FREE

Try not to overcook the beans. They should still have a bit of snap left when they get to the table!

1 pound fresh green beans, trimmed	½ teaspoon salt
½ cup water	⅛ teaspoon pepper
2 tablespoons white vinegar	¼ teaspoon dry mustard
	¼ teaspoon paprika

Place green beans in a saucepan. Combine remaining ingredients in a glass; pour over the beans. Simmer until hot.

Makes 4 servings

Green Beans Oregano

DAIRY-FREE
EGG-FREE
GLUTEN-FREE

Here's a quick trick to sauce up some fresh green beans while they are cooking. Test for tenderness and stop cooking as soon as they're crisp-tender.

1 pound fresh green beans, trimmed and cut
1 cup tomato juice
¼ teaspoon salt
¼ teaspoon oregano

Place beans in a heavy saucepan. Pour tomato juice over beans; add salt and oregano. Cook until beans are tender, about 15 minutes. Juice will thicken and become a flavorful sauce.

Makes 6 servings

Sweet and Sour Red Cabbage

DAIRY-FREE
EGG-FREE
GLUTEN-FREE

Sure, you like some grated red cabbage in your salad, and you've served it boiled now and then. But have you ever made a zingy sweet-and-sour-sauced offering? It's delicious.

1 medium head red cabbage shredded
1½ cups water
2 tablespoons brown sugar
2 tablespoons lemon juice
1 tablespoon wine vinegar
2 whole cloves
½ teaspoon ginger
½ teaspoon salt
⅛ teaspoon pepper

Place shredded cabbage in a deep saucepan. Add remaining ingredients and stir well. Cover and simmer 35 minutes, or until cabbage is tender.

Makes 6–8 servings

Pickled Cucumbers and Onions

DAIRY-FREE
EGG-FREE
GLUTEN-FREE

Add extra onion if you like and keep these pickled cukes in the refrigerator for several days at a time—if they last that long!

1 large or 2 small cucumbers
1 medium onion
½ cup white vinegar
¼ cup salad oil
1 teaspoon sugar
½ teaspoon salt
⅛ teaspoon pepper
¼ cup water

Pare cucumber and cut into paper-thin slices. Slice onion paper-thin and separate into rings. Place cucumber and onion in a small deep bowl or jar. Combine vinegar, oil, sugar, salt, and pepper; stir vigorously. Stir in water and immediately pour over cucumbers. Cover and refrigerate several hours or overnight.

Makes 4–6 servings

Vegetables with Peanut Sauce

DAIRY-FREE
EGG-FREE
GLUTEN-FREE

Here's an intriguing medley of vegetables that is held together by a divine sauce. Strictly for the adventurous palate!

2 cups water
1 pound fresh or 1 10-ounce package frozen leaf spinach
2 cups coarsely shredded cabbage
1 pound fresh or 1 10-ounce package frozen whole string beans
1 recipe Peanut Sauce (following recipe)

Bring water to a boil. Add vegetables, one at a time, and blanch each for 3–5 minutes. Drain. Bring water to a boil again before adding next vegetable. Combine vegetables in a serving bowl. Serve hot or at room temperature with Peanut Sauce.

Makes 6 servings

Peanut Sauce

1 tablespoon salad oil
¼ cup chopped onion
½ cup peanut butter
1 cup water
2 tablespoons pure soy sauce
⅛ teaspoon ground ginger
Dash of garlic powder
Dash of cayenne pepper

Heat salad oil in a heavy 1-quart saucepan over medium heat. Add onion and sauté until golden and transparent. Add peanut butter, stirring constantly. Gradually add water and soy sauce, stirring until smooth. Add ginger, garlic powder, and cayenne. Bring to a boil, stirring constantly, until sauce thickens. Pour over vegetables and serve.

Makes 1½ cups sauce

Stewed Tomatoes

DAIRY-FREE
EGG-FREE
GLUTEN-FREE

Go easy on the water, adding just enough to keep these tomatoes from sticking to the pot. It's not soup you're after!

6 tomatoes, washed and quartered
1 onion, sliced thin
½ teaspoon salt
¼ teaspoon pepper
1 teaspoon sugar
1 teaspoon lemon juice
½ cup water

Place tomatoes in a small heavy saucepan. Add sliced onion, salt, pepper, sugar, and lemon juice. Add water and cover tightly. Simmer for 20 minutes, stirring occasionally and adding more water if necessary to keep from sticking.

Makes 4 servings

Cherry Tomatoes Vinaigrette

DAIRY-FREE
EGG-FREE
GLUTEN-FREE

You'll want to serve these by the bowlful as a summer vegetable. They're packed with flavor!

¾ teaspoon salt
¼ teaspoon honey
¼ cup lemon juice
¾ cup salad oil
1 clove garlic, crushed
½ teaspoon dried basil
½ teaspoon dried thyme
1 tablespoon chopped parsley
2 pints cherry tomatoes

Combine salt, honey, lemon juice, salad oil, garlic, basil, thyme, and parsley in a bowl; mix well. Wash cherry tomatoes and remove stems. Add to dressing, mixing well. Chill at least 2 hours before serving.

Makes 6 servings

Tomato Aspic

DAIRY-FREE
EGG-FREE
GLUTEN-FREE

If you have never had real tomato aspic, give yourself a treat and make this one soon. It's so refreshing!

3 pounds fresh tomatoes
3 tablespoons lemon juice
2 tablespoons water
¼ cup chopped onion
¾ cup chopped celery
2 teaspoons sugar
1¼ teaspoons salt
½ teaspoon paprika
Dash of white pepper
1 bay leaf
1 teaspoon Worcestershire sauce
2 envelopes unflavored gelatin
⅓ cup cold water
Chicory and cucumber slices for garnish (optional)

Coarsely chop tomatoes (to make about 8 cups). Combine in a medium saucepan with lemon juice, 2 tablespoons water, onion, celery, sugar, salt, paprika, pepper, bay leaf, and Worcestershire sauce. Bring to a boil. Cover and simmer for 45 minutes. Strain tomato mixture, reserving liquid. Soften gelatin in ⅓ cup cold water in a small cup; place over boiling water and stir until dissolved. Stir gelatin mixture into strained tomato liquid. Pour into 6 individual ¾-cup molds. Chill until firm. Garnish with chicory and cucumber slices, if desired.

Makes 6 servings

Mixed Vegetable Casserole

DAIRY-FREE
EGG-FREE
GLUTEN-FREE

This casserole mixes a number of unforbidden foods beautifully—and flexibly. If someone is specifically sensitive to one of the ingredients, simply substitute it with a different vegetable.

2 potatoes, pared and cubed
2 carrots, pared and sliced
½ cauliflower, cut into flowerets
2 ribs celery, cut in slices
½ pound mushrooms, sliced
2 onions, sliced
1 red pepper, cut into strips
1 clove garlic, minced
1½ cups Chicken Broth (see recipe)
1 teaspoon pepper
2 teaspoons dried dillweed

Combine all ingredients in a 3-quart baking dish. Cover tightly and bake in a 350° F. oven for 1 hour, or until vegetables are tender.

Makes 8 servings

RICE

Pilau

DAIRY-FREE
EGG-FREE
GLUTEN-FREE

So you think cooked brown rice tastes dreary? Try it this way and thrill your taste buds tonight!

½ cup slivered almonds
¼ cup chopped pistachio nuts
2 tablespoons margarine
3 cups cooked brown rice (cooked in Chicken Broth, see recipe)
2 teaspoons ground mace

Sauté almonds and pistachio nuts in margarine about 3 minutes, stirring frequently. Add rice and mace. Heat thoroughly, tossing lightly to prevent sticking.

Makes 6 servings

Mushroom Rice Pilaf

DAIRY-FREE
EGG-FREE
GLUTEN-FREE

Cumin seed has a flavor all its own, but it's related to the parsley family and is often a part of curry and chili powders. Here it perks up a nice rice dish.

1 cup sliced onions
2 tablespoons dairy-free
  margarine
1 4-ounce can sliced
  mushrooms, drained
3 tablespoons chopped parsley
3 cups cooked brown rice
¼ teaspoon basil
½ teaspoon cumin seed

Cook onions in margarine until tender. Add remaining ingredients and heat thoroughly, stirring constantly.

Makes 6 servings

Carrot Rice Ring

DAIRY-FREE
EGG-FREE
GLUTEN-FREE

What a beautiful way to present a delicious combination! Fill the ring with cooked green vegetables for a color contrast.

3 cups fluffy cooked rice
2 cups chopped cooked carrots
½ cup white raisins
½ cup finely chopped fresh parsley
1 teaspoon salt
⅛ teaspoon pepper

Combine hot cooked rice, chopped cooked carrots, raisins, parsley, salt, and pepper. Pack firmly into a buttered 6-cup ring mold; let stand for 5 minutes and then turn out onto a serving platter.

Makes 6 servings

DESSERTS

Baked Apples

DAIRY-FREE
EGG-FREE
GLUTEN-FREE

Make extras of these baked apples as a ready dessert for those who can't have the family cake. These apples may be refrigerated for 3 to 4 days. No deprivation—these apples are a treat!

6 large baking apples
1 tablespoon brown sugar
⅓ cup golden raisins
½ teaspoon cinnamon
1 cup boiling water

Wash and core apples. Place in a flat baking dish. Combine brown sugar, raisins, and cinnamon. Fill cavity of each apple with this mixture. Pour boiling water around apples. Bake, uncovered, in a 350° F. oven for about 1 hour, or until tender. Occasionally baste apples with pan liquid.

Makes 6 servings

Applesauce Whip

DAIRY-FREE
EGG-FREE
GLUTEN-FREE

When there's a desire for a mouthful of fluffy goodness, try this scrumptious dessert. Try to use stemmed glasses for maximum effect.

1 1-tablespoon envelope unflavored gelatin
1 cup cold water
¼ cup sugar
2 tablespoons lemon juice
1 16-ounce can applesauce
¼ teaspoon cinnamon

Sprinkle gelatin over ½ cup of the water in a saucepan. Place over low heat; stir constantly until gelatin dissolves, about 3 minutes. Remove from heat. Stir in sugar, remaining ½ cup water, lemon juice, applesauce, and cinnamon. Chill, stirring occasionally until mixture is the consistency of unbeaten egg white. Beat with a rotary or electric mixer until light and fluffy. Spoon into individual dessert dishes and chill until set.

Makes 6 servings

Citrus Sherbet

DAIRY-FREE
EGG-FREE
GLUTEN-FREE

Allergies can make one suspicious of all store-bought sherbets. Here's the way to make your own and know just what's in it!

3 cups water
1 cup light corn syrup
1 tablespoon grated lemon
  rind

¾ cup sugar
1 envelope unflavored gelatin
⅔ cup lemon juice
½ cup orange juice

Mix together water, corn syrup, sugar, and lemon rind in a large, heavy saucepan. Cook over medium heat, stirring constantly, until sugar is dissolved and mixture comes to a boil. Boil 5 minutes. Remove from heat. Meanwhile, sprinkle gelatin over lemon juice to soften; add to hot mixture and stir until gelatin is dissolved. Add orange juice. Cool to lukewarm. Strain, if desired. Pour into a 9-by-5-inch loaf pan and freeze 3–4 hours, or until mixture is firm. Turn into a large chilled bowl. Beat until smooth and fluffy but not melted. Wash and dry the loaf pan before filling with mixture. Freeze about 3½ hours or until firm.

Makes 12 servings

Fruit Juice Gelatin

DAIRY-FREE
EGG-FREE
GLUTEN-FREE

Here's an easy way to make your own gelatin. If sugar in the diet is limited, omit in this recipe.

1 envelope unflavored gelatin
½ cup cold water
¼ cup sugar
1½ cups fruit juice (any choice but fresh or
    frozen pineapple juice)

Sprinkle gelatin over water in a small saucepan. Place over low heat; stir constantly until gelatin dissolves, about 3 minutes. Remove from heat. Stir in sugar. Stir in juice. Pour into 4 individual dishes or a 2-cup mold. Chill until set.

Makes 4 servings

NOTE: To add fruit to gelatin, use 1¼ cups fruit juice and chill until slightly thickened. Then add 1½ cups cut-up fresh, frozen, or canned fruit (except fresh or frozen pineapple) and pour into 6 individual dishes or a 3-cup mold. Chill until set.

Makes 6 servings

Dried Fruit Compote

DAIRY-FREE
EGG-FREE
GLUTEN-FREE

This can be served as dessert or as a side dish with roast beef. Either way, you'll get rave reviews for the effort.

1½ pounds mixed dried fruits, such as prunes, apricots, and pears	1 tablespoon grated lemon rind
Cold water	½ teaspoon cinnamon
2 tablespoons brown sugar	⅛ teaspoon nutmeg
2 tablespoons honey	2 tablespoons cornstarch
	¼ cup orange juice

Cover dried fruits with cold water and let stand at room temperature for several hours or overnight. Drain off water and measure 1 cup of it to pour into a saucepan. Add sugar, honey, lemon rind, cinnamon, and nutmeg. Bring to a boil and cook for 5 minutes. Mix cornstarch and orange juice together until smooth; stir into pan. Add drained fruits; stir until sauce is thickened and fruit is hot. Can also be cooled and served cold.

Makes 8 servings

Poached Oranges

DAIRY-FREE
EGG-FREE
GLUTEN-FREE

Here's how to turn an ordinary orange into an extraordinary dessert. Read the margarine label carefully to be sure that dried milk solids are not included in the product.

6 oranges
3 tablespoons nondairy
   margarine
¾ cup currant jelly

½ cup orange juice
1 tablespoon cornstarch
2 tablespoons cold water

Remove thin outer rind from three of the oranges, using a vegetable peeler, and cut into very thin slivers. Place rind in a small saucepan, cover with water, and bring to a boil; reduce heat and simmer for 10 minutes. Drain, reserving rind. Cut remaining rind and white membrane from all 6 oranges. Place margarine and currant jelly into a large skillet; cook and stir until melted. Stir in orange juice and reserved cooked slivered rind. Add oranges and simmer for 5 minutes, spooning sauce over oranges as they poach. Combine cornstarch and cold water to form a smooth paste; add some of the orange sauce and then return all to the skillet, stirring until smooth. Cook until mixture bubbles and thickens, continuing to spoon sauce over oranges. Serve warm, covered with sauce.

Makes 6 servings

Coconut Cookies

DAIRY-FREE
EGG-FREE
GLUTEN-FREE

It is almost impossible to bake without flour, milk, and eggs, but here's a cookie that does it very nicely.

⅓ cup brown sugar
¼ cup shortening
1 teaspoon pure vanilla
  extract
¼ cup orange juice

1 cup cornstarch
1½ teaspoons baking powder
¼ teaspoon salt
2 tablespoons shredded
  coconut

Beat sugar and shortening together until fluffy. Add vanilla extract. Alternately add orange juice and mixture of cornstarch, baking powder, salt, and coconut. Form into a log of dough by rolling in waxed paper. Chill for 1 hour. Cut cookies ¼ inch thick and place on a greased baking sheet. Bake in a preheated 375° F. oven for about 25 minutes, or until edges are lightly browned.

Makes about 1½ dozen

Peanut Butter Popcorn

DAIRY-FREE
EGG-FREE
GLUTEN-FREE

If there is no allergy to corn, here's a good, crunchy treat.

3 quarts freshly popped corn
1 cup sugar
⅔ cup light corn syrup
⅔ cup chunky peanut butter
1 teaspoon vanilla
½ teaspoon baking soda

Place popcorn in a large, shallow roasting pan. In a heavy 1½-quart saucepan, stir together sugar and corn syrup. Stirring constantly, cook over medium heat until mixture boils. Stir in peanut butter. Continue cooking, without stirring, for 5 minutes. Remove from heat. Stir in vanilla and baking soda. Pour peanut butter mixture over popcorn. Stir to coat well. Bake in a low (250° F.) oven, stirring occasionally, for 1 hour. Turn into another large roasting pan to cool, stirring occasionally to break apart. Store in a tightly covered container.

Makes 3 quarts

APPENDIX
Sample Menu for the
Dairy-Free/Egg-Free/Gluten-Free Diet*

The dairy-free, egg-free, gluten-free diet is the most difficult to follow. Instead of concentrating on the foods you cannot serve, it is best to write down menus of what can be eaten. Here is a sample of two such days to show you that it can be done deliciously and nutritiously.

Breakfast
Apple juice
Cooked grits with margarine and raisins
    (thin with soy milk or water)
Herbal tea or allowable beverage

Lunch
Tomato juice
Herbed Hamburgers
Cooked carrots
Fresh spinach salad
Fruit Juice Gelatin
Herbal tea or allowable beverage

---

*All recipes in italic can be found in the index.

Dinner
  Vegetable Soup
  Chicken Italienne
  Rice Pilau
  Zesty Green Beans
  Fresh green salad
  Citrus Sherbet
  Herbal tea or allowable beverage

Breakfast
  Orange juice
  Cold rice cereal with pineapple juice
  Banana (may be sliced in the cereal, if desired)
  Herbal tea or allowable beverage

Lunch
  Boiled Salmon
  Stewed Tomatoes
  Corn on the cob
  Fresh Fruit Salad
  Herbal tea or allowable beverage

Dinner
  Pea Soup
  Flank Steak Teriyaki
  Baked potato
  Broccoli with margarine
  Fresh green salad
  Baked Apple
  Herbal tea or allowable beverage

Index

As you look through this index, notice the symbols DF, EF, and GF that follow each recipe. Through these symbols, you can tell at a glance whether or not any recipe is appropriate for your cooking needs.

- DF stands for dairy-free. If you or someone for whom you are cooking is allergic to dairy products, use this recipe. It calls for no dairy products.
- EF stands for egg-free. If you or someone for whom you are cooking is allergic to eggs, use this recipe. It calls for no eggs.
- GF stands for gluten-free. If you or someone for whom you are cooking is allergic to gluten flours, use this recipe. It calls for no gluten flours.

A combination of symbols means that a recipe is free from all allergens listed. Thus "EF, GF" after a recipe name indicates that the recipe is *both* egg-free and gluten-free.